SpringerBriefs in Public Health

SpringerBriefs in Public Health present concise summaries of cutting-edge research and practical applications from across the entire field of public health, with contributions from medicine, bioethics, health economics, public policy, biostatistics, and sociology.

The focus of the series is to highlight current topics in public health of interest to a global audience, including health care policy; social determinants of health; health issues in developing countries; new research methods; chronic and infectious disease epidemics; and innovative health interventions.

Featuring compact volumes of 50 to 125 pages, the series covers a range of content from professional to academic. Possible volumes in the series may consist of timely reports of state-of-the art analytical techniques, reports from the field, snapshots of hot and/or emerging topics, elaborated theses, literature reviews, and in-depth case studies. Both solicited and unsolicited manuscripts are considered for publication in this series.

Briefs are published as part of Springer's eBook collection, with millions of users worldwide. In addition, Briefs are available for individual print and electronic purchase.

Briefs are characterized by fast, global electronic dissemination, standard publishing contracts, easy-to-use manuscript preparation and formatting guidelines, and expedited production schedules. We aim for publication 8–12 weeks after acceptance.

More information about this series at http://www.springer.com/series/10138

Thomas F. Hilton • Carl G. Leukefeld

Grantsmanship for New Investigators

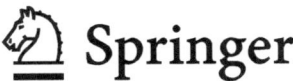 Springer

Thomas F. Hilton (Retired)
Indian Harbour Beach, FL, USA

Carl G. Leukefeld
School of Medicine
Center on Drug and Alcohol Research
University of Kentucky
Lexington, KY, USA

ISSN 2192-3698   ISSN 2192-3701   (electronic)
SpringerBriefs in Public Health
ISBN 978-3-030-01300-4   ISBN 978-3-030-01301-1   (eBook)
https://doi.org/10.1007/978-3-030-01301-1

Library of Congress Control Number: 2018958645

This Springer imprint is published by the registered company Springer Nature Switzerland AG
The registered company address is: Gewerbestrasse 11, 6330 Cham, Switzerland

To Frank Tims, Ph.D., friend, mentor, and scholar, whose work over many decades has advanced the careers of so many scientists in health services research

Contents

About the Authors

Over the span of more than four decades, both Tom Hilton and Carl Leukefeld have worked as bench and field researchers as well as federal grant and contract administrators at various federal agencies including the world's largest grantor, the National Institutes of Health (NIH). Tom's career has focused on applied research and grants administration in mostly nonacademic roles, whereas over half of Carl's career as a public health researcher has been spent in academic settings.

Tom Hilton is a retired Navy captain and a retired industrial/organizational psychologist. While a pre- and postdoctoral fellow at the Institute of Behavioral Research, Tom's work involved drafting applications and conducting both grant and contract research projects for the Departments of Defense, Transportation, and Health and Human Services. Projects also involved county, state, and private sector organizations. In 1979, Tom joined the psychiatry faculty at Southwestern Medical School where he started a small lab evaluating public health services after winning his first grant from a private foundation. In 1982, Tom was recalled to active Navy duty to lead research projects in shipboard and hospital health services delivery systems and later oversaw Navy's applied personnel and training research programs at the Pentagon. Spanning much of his Navy career, Tom served on Office of Naval Research grant and contract review panels. In 1992, Tom became the founding manager of a Federal Aviation Administration laboratory studying employee development, process improvement, and personnel selection. Coincident with that role, he also completed a 3-year detail to the White House Office of Reinventing Government until 2000 when he retired from the Navy and joined the National Institute on Drug Abuse at NIH. Until his retirement in 2012, Tom served on the NIH extramural faculty that trains new grant program officials, the advisory group for NIH grants administration IT systems, and science officer for a 9-year research project involving all 28 NIH institutes and centers. Over the years, Tom has attended hundreds of grant and contract proposal review meetings, and he has served as project officer for many of the grants and contracts that were funded. He has 56 refereed publications and has presented over 80 papers, symposia, and professional development workshops.

Carl Leukefeld is Professor of Behavioral Science and Psychiatry as well as Chair of the Department of Behavioral Science and founding Director of the Center on Drug and Alcohol Research at the University of Kentucky. He is also the Bell Alcohol and Addictions Endowed Chair. He joined the University of Kentucky in 1990 to establish the Center on Drug and Alcohol Research from the National Institute on Drug Abuse (NIDA) where he held administrative and research positions including grant and contract planning, developing requests for applications and proposals, grant reviews, developing grant review summary statements, and research project administration. He was also the Chief Health Services Officer of the United States Public Health Service. Carl's external grant support experience includes funded grants from NIH, NSF, as well as contracts from states, community organizations, and industry. Carl has also served as a reviewer and consulting journal editor, ad hoc grant reviewer for federal agencies like the CDC and NIH, and has been a standing member of National Institutes of Health initial review groups (IRG) – sometimes referred to as study sections. In addition to workshops and courses on grant preparation, he has taught undergraduate, graduate, and medical students. His publications include over 350 articles, chapters, books, and monographs.

Introduction

What This Book Is

This brief book introduces readers to grantsmanship by discussing strategies that will help you put forth the best argument for funding your research project. We focus on the National Institutes of Health application process because it is the most comprehensive of all grant review and administrative systems. With an annual budget of over $68 billion, NIH dwarfs all other sources of external research funding globally. As such, most funding institutions, public or private, tend to model their systems and procedures after NIH. We will touch on some notable differences between NIH and other agencies and funders that may affect how you decide to approach them.

There are many grantsmanship books available which describe rules, regulations, and application procedures. Unfortunately, they tend to be long on description but short on helping you understand how to work the process to your advantage. We hope this book fills that niche in the grantsmanship literature.

We apply our combined eight-plus decades of experience as researchers; grant and contract applicants; application reviewers; and contract, grant, and research program administrators in Academia, DOD, DOT, HHS, and the private sector to highlight ways in which new investigators can help convince targeted funding institutions that their research project is worthy of support. Specifically, we hope you will learn more about:

- Identifying factors to consider when exploring funding options for your project
- Understanding available grant mechanisms for new investigators
- Understanding what is involved in pursuing federal support, including common misconceptions
- Building your entire career using grant support
- Thinking strategically throughout the application process (not just before formal submission)
- Understanding ideal ways to describe your project when completing application forms

- Understanding the peer technical review process
- Identifying strategies for responding to concerns if you are not funded or funding is deferred
- Appreciating the grant vetting process and identifying ways to increase your odds of funding once your project has been favorably reviewed

What This Book Is Not

This book is not a cookbook, nor is it an official procedural manual or even a comprehensive description of the grants process. Some policies and procedures we mention may be revised before this book is even published. Government agencies continually try to improve procedures or modify them to meet new legislation. We have overlooked a few nuanced topics not because we were unaware of them necessarily but because new investigators are unlikely to encounter them or are well-prepared to address them.

We encourage all grant applicants to read published grant and contract Funding Opportunity Announcements (FOAs) carefully. Each government and private sector institution's FOA will specify required information, forms, formats, and the submission system to use when applying for their grants or contracts. Go to the websites of your target funding institutions to learn more about their general mission focus and to clarify any specific requirements that were unclear in the FOA.

Chapter 1
Exploring Funding Options

Tactics are things done to advance one's position. Strategies are how you integrate those tactics to achieving your ultimate objective. That objective, in this book, is obtaining research funding. Thus, **we emphasize strategic thinking throughout the book.** The more you know about grants and contracts, as well as agencies and foundations; the better equipped you are to engage in grantsmanship. Understanding how applications are prepared, assembled, submitted, peer reviewed, and vetted for funding; you can organize your application in ways to avoid common mistakes while positively influencing application reviewers.

1.1 Is the Federal Government Giving Away Free Money?

Matthew Lesko is a guy who for decades appeared on night-owl TV dressed in a suit covered in question marks telling viewers that the "Federal Government is Giving Away Free Money!" He reminded the audience that they would be "crazy to miss this opportunity." Mr. Lesko is somewhat retired today, but his message is not as crazy as he often acted. Every year, the US federal government does award billions of dollars (over $68BN in 2016) to fund research across a broad variety of agencies.

Perspective of the Government Of course, a research grant is not really a gift and is certainly not an entitlement. From the government's perspective awarding a grant is **using tax dollars to buy (fund) the best science** in order to answer questions that will advance the health, welfare, and safety of its citizens. In so doing, grants help to promote the economic growth of the nation and advance scientific knowledge.

To achieve these aims, agencies must have staff with the relevant scientific expertise to administer, review, vet, fund, and monitor compliance with federal rules and regulations. Each agency has an office responsible for grants and contracts adminis-

© The Author(s), under exclusive license to Springer Nature Switzerland AG 2019
T. F. Hilton, C. G. Leukefeld, *Grantsmanship for New Investigators*,
SpringerBriefs in Public Health, https://doi.org/10.1007/978-3-030-01301-1_1

tration which also has to have expert staff to ensure applicant eligibility and compliance with government rules and regulations that protect humans, animals, and the interests of the taxpayers on whose behalf the grant was issued. Staff also gauge responsiveness to federal announcements and ensure grant/contract awardees are using appropriate scientific methods.

Perspective of the Applicant From the applicant's perspective, applying for a grant is like running in a marathon. It gets easier after each competition – win or lose. Thus, submitting a grant application requires a serious time-commitment that includes thoroughly studying the requirements of the agency's funding opportunity announcement (FOA)[1] to determine their organization's eligibility, capacity, structure, and resource availability to meet the purpose of the grant; obtain commitments from the researcher's institution to apply if appropriate, arrange for a lab, other equipment and other infrastructure; recruit a research team; identify a fruitful approach to recruit research subjects, determine how human subjects will be protected or how other sources of data will be accessed; obtain letters of commitment to provide access to subjects and/or other research materials in event the grant is awarded, and develop a budget within federal guidelines to cover the cost of completing the project. A principal investigator (PI) must have a command of the research literature; identify gaps in the science; write; edit, proof; and submit an application, or have it electronically submitted before the specified due date (deadline). That is a tall order.

1.2 Why Apply for Grants?

According to the National Institutes of Health (NIH), the odds of being awarded one of their grants are about 1 in 4 (Rockley 2016; GAO 2015). Although that sounds high, these odds are far better than Las Vegas odds or winning a lottery. Also, the size of the US Federal jackpot (award) is considerably more attractive than most other sources of research support. Compare the US's $68BN/year research budget to that of the European Union Research Council (ERC) which is less than $2BN/year.[2] Even factoring in domestic research support among European Union members, the US dwarfs other countries.[3]

   There is no debating the fact that it takes creativity, motivation, time, and effort to successfully prepare a federal research application. As the saying goes, "Time is money." Therefore, federal research grants are not exactly "free" in any sense of the word. This is especially true considering that it is not unusual to repeat this cycle of

---

[1] Appendix E list the majority of acronyms used in the alphabet soup of grantsmanship.

[2] The 6-year budget for the European Research Council (ERC) is $13.6 BN, or about $2BN/year (downloaded from https://erc.europa.eu/about-erc/facts-and-figures on 06/05/2018). Formed in 2007, ERC is the European Union's equivalent of the US NIH and NSF combined.

[3] China and Russia sometimes claim a larger research investment than the US, but when looking at the basis for their claims, they factor in industrial research and development activities that are excluded from the US federally-supported basic and applied research budget.

activities 2–4 times before a grant application is funded. Worse, there is always the possibility that the project will never attract a buyer.

So, what is the motivation to compete for federal research grants? What is the payoff? There are four major reasons why any researcher would be motivated to pursue a grant application even if there is not a 100% chance of getting funded. These include:

(a) Career enhancement – academic recognition, prestige and promotion,
(b) Financial support for you and your students,
(c) Freedom to creatively follow your idea and the data,
(d) Knowledge to successfully bridge to entrepreneurial success.

1.2.1 Career Enhancement: Academic Recognition, Prestige and Promotion

Like any private or public-sector researcher, academic promotions go to leaders in their field. Grant and contract support is important to institutions because it funds indirect costs such as overhead, graduate student support, salary for faculty and research staff, and it brings prestige to the grantee institution. Leadership includes peer-reviewed research publications that influence the direction of colleagues. Also, for non-academic researchers, success often entails winning repeat business for contracts.

In academic settings, a dissertation or fellowship grant can demonstrate to selection committees that an applicant for a tenure-track faculty position has the potential for getting future funding. Some recent PhDs are not landing tenure-track positions, leaving them to start their careers on the margins of academic research (e.g., Jaschik 2009; Larson et al. 2014; Finder 2007). Even after getting a research or tenure-track position, faculty are still only on the "track" to tenure. Faculty usually do not get tenure until they have published a minimum number of refereed papers, and that usually requires grant or contract research support. Similarly, the track to full professor is increasingly tied to income-producing research. The really big guns on campus, the institute directors, are grant heavy-hitters who bring in millions of dollars each year that support faculty colleagues, post-docs, and graduate students. In addition, there are endowed chairs and professorships, which pay an above-the-norm salary for those leaders. Even though some endowed chairs have a guaranteed salary, most endowed chairs and professors were offered their positions because of their long history of grant awards.

1.2.2 Financial Support for You and Your Students

Grants normally provide indirect costs including overhead, salaries, and benefits – sometimes equipment and facilities. Grants often enable academics to "buy" their way out of teaching classes in order to free up time for their research. Funding also might be a way to stay in academia without a tenure-track position such as a research professor working in a university-based institute. Of course, because research professors live on "soft money" (from grant to grant), they have to sustain their positions by bringing grants and contracts into their institute or risk seeing their support dry up. After a period of consistently bringing money into the institute, most research professors are eventually awarded salaried, tenured positions.

A big plus associated with grant awards can be support for graduate students. For example, Tom's doctoral work was supported by both federal grants and corporate contracts. His fellowship grants waived tuition, and contract support helped to pay for living expenses. Of greater value, was Tom's on-the-job, supervised experience, that not only helped to hone research skills, but also to learn how to market research and use results to improve agency mission accomplishment or company profitability. On the other hand, Carl's doctoral work was supported by the National Institute of Mental Health as a fellow which did not require work on specific studies.

Many universities will only accept a student into their doctoral programs if they can be supported through their major professor's grants and contracts. Thus, your grants and contract income usually means that you get to choose the students with whom you will work. Their success can help them compete independently for dissertation grants and post-docs thereby enabling you to support additional students.

1.2.3   Freedom to Creatively Follow Your Ideas and the Data

Grants   One of the best aspects of government grants is that you do not have a task master. Once your grant is awarded, you as PI have wide latitude in its execution. You may add variables not in the application so that you can address a wider range of hypotheses and/or help your students collect dissertation data. You can also change the sample somewhat. But – you may not spend more money than your total grant award, and, you must test all hypotheses listed in your application – unless you have arranged for alternative testing with your funding institution's Project Officer (PO). It is strongly recommended that you discuss significant post-award changes with your funding organization's PO. Keeping your funding agency POs and contract officers informed will help to ensure their continued support should unforeseen problems arise such as costly equipment failure or an adverse event affecting subjects.

Funding latitude is particularly welcome when your data start to suggest that the answers to questions emerging from the data are not in the current design. Because grants are often awarded for 3–5 years, there might be enough time to replicate, enroll additional subjects, merge your data with that of a colleague, and other activities that let you follow where the data take you. Your funding institution PO might even supplement your award to enable you to do those things. On a variety of occasions, both Tom and Carl convinced their institute directors to award supplemental funds or contracts when justified by emerging results.

Of course, not all grants offer funding latitude. When that is the case, it is normally specified in federal funding opportunity announcements (FOAs). For example, this is sometimes the case when agencies need an extramural project to supplement their own intramural research. Because others are depending on your research deliverables, these kinds of grants (usually modest) add needed expertise (yours) to ensure the success of a larger project.

Contracts The Department of Defense (DOD), the Department of Transportation (DOT – especially the Federal Aviation Administration), and the National Aeronautics and Space Administration rely heavily on the contract mechanism to support their research needs. This is in part because these agencies support large intramural research organizations of their own, and as such, may only need outside expertise for a specific part of a project. It is important to underscore the idea that very few contracts offer the funding latitude provided by grants. In fact, contract awards are often modified post-award. During Tom's military career, it was not uncommon to reprogram funds for one contract to initiate a new high-priority study. This was rationalized by extending the length of cut projects (i.e., stretching the initial award into the next fiscal year).

When latitude is viewed to be advantageous to the government, contracts are usually referred to as "cost-plus," which means changes requested by the government that drive up the cost are chargeable in addition to the original contract award. Such "Plus-ups" normally require approval by the Contracting Officer (CO), the federal official overseeing the project (as recommended by the Contracting Officer's Technical Representative – COTR). Relatively few bench scientists will ever be directly involved in cost-plus work. Most cost-plus research contracts tend to go to large companies and corporations like Boeing, Harris, Northrop-Grumman, and Lockheed Martin that are capable of building things like nuclear submarines, fighter jets, and rocket ships.

All federal agencies may contract for research projects that might appeal to bench scientists with special expertise. Some of these relatively smaller, briefer contracts are competed like grants, while others are sole-sourced. To win a sole-source contract, you and your lab must be renowned for special expertise that is either scarce in the world, or because you have extensive familiarity with funding institution systems (often through prior grants and contracts), and/or have government security clearances, that are key to timely execution.

1.2.4   Springboard to Entrepreneurial Success

Federally funded research can lead to the discovery of new technology. Inventions developed from federally funded research projects are required to be reported to the government agency that funded the project, per the Bayh-Dole Act (the Patent and Trademark Law Amendments Act of 1980). With the exception of the Defense Department, most grants allow the investigator to take title to any inventions if the

PI or the PI's organization intend to market them. However, the government retains license rights forever. Usually that means the government can use the invention at its discretion, and you cannot sue it for patent infringement.

Generally, federal grants can be a launching pad for new businesses. In fact, all federal agencies offer grants to conduct research and development to attract capital investment called Small Business Innovative Research Grants (SBIRs) or Science Technology Transfer Research Grants (STTRs). For example, Medimmune in Gaithersburg Maryland, which develops vaccines and therapeutic drugs, started on NIH grant money. Of course, you may have a contract clause with your employer or university, which gives them certain rights. But there is no question that federal research grants can be a springboard to entrepreneurial success. Why? The federal government is eager to encourage the use of research findings to expand its economy and otherwise improve the public's welfare.

1.3 Winning, Even on an Uneven Playing Field

With the odds being 1 in 4 or worse, it might seem like the field of competition for grants is not an even playing field. It isn't. Grant competition is an uphill playing field. However, you can improve your odds of winning an award. For example, senior PIs rarely compete for small grants. Thus, small grant applicants tend to be competing with people of similar experience. Over time, PIs compete for bigger and bigger projects building on prior successes. Although the review process is fair, the NIH vetting process following peer review, weighs publications, experience, etc. when making funding decisions among similarly scored projects, and handicaps highly-experienced applicants to encourage tomorrow's top researchers.

You should expect things to be more arduous at first because you face mountains of unfamiliar rules, are unsure how the referees (senior colleagues) will score your application in review, and you are likely competing with a few proven stars in your field. Nevertheless, your doctoral training, especially the dissertation process, provides supervised experience in proposing, executing, and presenting findings to an audience of senior colleagues. You might not have been thinking about that phase of your training as a grants boot camp, but it was.

It is sometimes said that the "P" in PhD stands for persistence. We doubt that anybody reading this would disagree. Persistence is also how you successfully compete for grant awards. NIH's own analyses show that **many new investigators give up after only one or two applications**, thus improving the odds for the persistent (Heggeness et al. 2016). Of course, not all grant applicants can afford to be persistent. Some are on soft money that runs out before they get a grant to cover their salary.

Nevertheless, we learn from our failures as well as successes, so the odds of successfully competing for grants usually improve over time. A study by Matthews, Calhoun Lo, and Ho (2011) reported that between 1980 and 2008, the average age of the most prestigious R01 research project grants at NIH had increased by almost

12 years. So, yes, experience is a big plus. Of course, several factors contribute to such results. With no mandated retirements, some PIs are working into their late 70s. Like Carl, these senior researchers have well-established positions of leadership both within their organizations and within their fields. They work with experienced research teams and can offer settings and laboratories with the latest equipment. That experience makes them formidable competitors.

This age effect has led to complaints about a good-ole-boy system that virtually excludes new investigators. Things are more complex than that, but there is no denying that review panels are comprised of senior colleagues. Regardless, studies continue to find no systematic evidence of peer review unfairness.

Encouraging News! In an effort to ensure that the review system does not inadvertently discourage young talent and novel ideas, NIH took the initiative to institute a special handicapping system to advantage first-time (new investigator) and early-career applicants.[4]

You do NOT have to apply for "new investigator (NI)" status because NIH knows if you have previously been awarded a grant. However, you must input information into NIH's system to gain "Early Stage Investigator (ESI)" status (less than 10 years from your terminal doctorate). What is the difference between NI's and ESI's? <u>An NI has never before had a significant research grant regardless of career stage. ESI's are NI's who are less than 10 years out of school</u> (including residencies). NI's get a little slack during peer review and award vetting. ESI's get a bit more slack. How much latitude an NI or ESI is given usually depends on the budget and review percentile. Although once a researcher is awarded a first significant grant (normally an R01), they permanently lose their NI status. However, what successful new investigators do not lose, is the competitive advantage derived from a successful application experience and the professional momentum from their own funded research.

Recently, NIH ESI policy got criticized for overlooking younger mid-career investigators, so NIH recently came up with the Mid-Career Investigator status for those within 10 years of receiving their first NIH R01. The goal remains lowering the average age of R01 recipients overall. Will this work? Time will tell.

There are also "New Innovator Awards" (DP2) and "Early Independence Awards" (DP5) for gifted applicants. "Gifted" means highly productive as a pre-doc, and 5 recommendations from faculty and leaders in the field attesting to your potential. DP2s require little but proof that your profs think you are a genius, but DP2s only offer $1.5 M over 5 years to tinker. DP5 applicants must be predoctoral with anticipated completion within 12 months of the application submission. These are highly competitive grants of up to $250 K/year for 5 years (like a typical R01). However, fewer awards are made NIH-wide annually. If you are a genius, go for it!

---

[4]If you have Co-PIs listed, all of them must qualify for ESI status to get special consideration because this program is to encourage independent investigators.

1.4   Eligibility: Who May Apply for Government Grants?

Any US citizen or organization/institution may apply for a federal grant. However, **nearly all research grants are given to institutions**; not to individuals, not even to Nobel Laureates.[5] There are four main reasons for that: accountability, bureaucracy, talent, and costs.

Accountability Congress realizes that it may be questioned by the voters about the way tax money is being spent. Therefore, Congress has passed laws, which agencies turn into regulations that govern the behavior of grant recipients. For example, there are rules and regulations affecting human protection, animal protection, environmental protection, even how much salary compensation is allowed. There are also rules about who owns discoveries including a patentable process, device, or medication.

Bureaucracy You can imagine that holding every individual grantee accountable for hundreds of regulations would take an army of bureaucrats the size of, well, the Army! By giving funds to universities and other institutions, the system almost governs itself through funded agency responsibility. Noncompliance risks forfeiture of not only one researcher's grant money, but also all federal grant and contract funding the institution receives – not to mention fines. That creates quite an incentive for following the rules. In addition, Congress wants to know that if they ever inquire about a funded research project, the federal funding agency can answer their questions. This requires a large group of federal research project officers (PO's) to administer the federal monies awarded. Thus, in NIH, as in most agencies, Program Officials/Program Directors (same role different titles) responsible for administering national programs of research, take on the role of project officers (again POs) once an application becomes a funded grant in their portfolio of projects.

Talent Like the bank robber who robs banks because that's where the money is, the government awards grants to universities and research institutions because that is where the talented researchers are. The PI (Principal Investigator) for a research project is an important "factor" in grant competition. Your aunt Martha might have a swell idea for curing cancer, but her basement laboratory and master's degree in history is unlikely to be rated as qualifying for a grant during peer review. Thus, education and history of achievement, including leadership in the appropriate field of a study, is a significant factor affecting which applicants will be most qualified to carry out their proposed project. As mentioned earlier, offices that receive federal grant applications such as NIH's Office of Extramural Research also serve as clearinghouses. They screen each application and only forward to peer review those that meet eligibility qualifications.

---

[5] There are a few exceptions such as dissertation grants and fellowship grants.

Costs Aside from regulatory compliance, there is another reason for awarding grants to institutions. When institutions already have most of the talent and infra-structure to execute their proposed research, the amount requested is usually more competitive (smaller). Cost might be a tie-breaker for applicants competing for similar projects – especially Research Project Grant Requests for Application (RPG RFAs) or their contract equivalent Requests for Proposals (RFPs) which specify a fixed cost ceiling with a brief application time-window. Even if there is no immedi-ate competitor during a review cycle, a high price tag might cause the funding agency/institute to defer (put off) a funding decision to see if a more meritorious unsolicited program RPG application appears in the next review cycle. Deferral frees funds for other awards for the immediate cycle. When a deferral occurs, appli-cants may exercise some grantsmanship by trying to negotiate with the assigned agency PO for a lower cost by eliminating some tasks or by finding sponsors to co-fund the project with the primary funding agency.

1.5   What Research Support Is Available: The Three F's

There are three main sources of funds for basic and applied research. We call them the Three F's: Faculty Research Funds, Foundations, and the Federal Government.

Faculty Research Funds Of the three, Faculty Research Funds, often referred to as intramural research grants, offer fewest resources, but also the most latitude to take risks. Faculty intramural research is often the crucible of cutting-edge sci-ence – projects for which there is insufficient evidence to convince an extramural agency that the project will likely succeed. Faculty Research Funds are most often used as a springboard for new faculty to build a case for "extramural" research grant applications. However, sometimes established faculty need funds for a pilot project aimed at breaking new ground.

Where does the money come from for intramural faculty research? Some Faculty Research Funds come in the form of federal institutional research development grants intended to strengthen a school or department's research capabilities. Institutions apply for the grants and then are given the discretion to select which student(s) or faculty member(s) are most worthy. Additional funds can come from institutionally-related foundations, bequests, and donations.

Foundations Foundations are institutions that typically fund small to medium sized projects that are stepping stones to implementing breakthrough science such as the MacArthur Foundation, Bill & Melinda Gates Foundation, or Robert Wood Johnson Foundation. They sometimes help supplement large federal projects which overlap with their mission. An example might be the National Cancer Society con-tributing support to an NIH National Cancer Institute RPG. With few exceptions, the endowment of most foundations is too applied or too small or their mission focus is too narrow to independently support large research projects. For example, when Carl and Tom were at NIH, they periodically invited collaborative funding support for meritorious projects too pricey for their institute to justify. By partnering with a foundation, federal POs can help to lower the cost to the government to make a riskier or more-costly project more competitive for federal funding.

You can find out more about foundations that might fund your area of research at *The Foundation Center* (foundationcenter.org), which maintains a comprehensive database on U.S. and global grant-makers and their funding opportunities. A great way to learn about foundations is from colleagues who have had experience with a foundation. Many foundations have very informal application processes. Review might be conducted by a single officer or by a board of directors. Some might be more focused on the science, while others might be more concerned about the impact on the public or their constituency. As a rule of thumb, the bigger the foundation; the bigger the grants, and the more it functions like NIH.

Federal Government As previously noted, the US federal government has the deepest pockets in the world when it comes to buying academic research. The government funds projects that might require several years to complete and cost millions of dollars. When there is strong Congressional encouragement or pressing public need, agencies have committed to projects taking a decade or more and hundreds of millions of dollars to complete. The NIH Human Genome Project is a high-profile example. It cost $2.7 billion dollars. Involved numerous research institutions and took more than a dozen years. While projects like that are rare by virtue of their cost and impact on resources, they serve to demonstrate that federal grants are the major leagues when it comes to research funding.

Keep in mind that each federal agency is trying to buy the best research with the highest likelihood that it will positively impact the public. Thus, the government does not buy a lot of cutting edge, risky, research that might never pan out. **The government buys safe research.** We will discuss more about the role played by research risk in Chap. 6 when we address application review.

1.6   Grants Versus Contracts

Throughout this book, we focus on grants rather than contracts because a) new investigators rarely rely upon contracts early in their careers, and b) the application development, review, and vetting processes for contracts are similar to those for grants. We also focus on NIH grants and contracts because, as Fig. 1.1 demonstrates, the NIH research budget dwarfs all other federal agencies even the Defense Department (DOD). Thus, if you understand how NIH processes grant and contract applications, you can anticipate that grantsmanship strategies recommended in this book are likely to be effective regardless of the funding institution to which you apply.

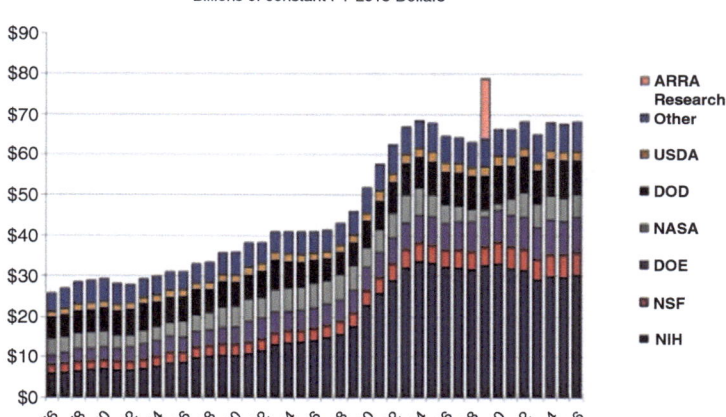

Trends in Research by Agency, FY 1976-2016
Billions of constant FY 2015 Dollars

Source: 1976-1994 figures are from the NSF federal funds survey; remainder is from AAASR&D reports.
FY 2015 are estimates, FY2016 is the President's request. © 2015 AAAS

Fig. 1.1 Graph showing US research investments between 1976 and 2016 broken down by major funding agency (White House Office of Science & Technology, 2013). Republished with permission of the American Association for the Advancement of Science (AAAS). (Source: AAAS Report: Research & Development series and analyses of FY 2018 omnibus legislation. https://www.aaas.org/sites/default/files/Agencies;.jpg)

However, contracts differ in ways that researchers need to consider, which is the purpose of this section. Federal, state, and municipal research contracts are frequently awarded to augment an agency's intramural research programs. As such, contract research often produces a component part of somebody else's project. Contract research is usually a primary business line, and as such, the contracted performing organization is usually in the private sector, and usually has an established relationship with both public and private sector customers. When universities are contracted, it is usually because they are a known and established center of excellence that engages in projects, which, for example, involve sophisticated engineering processes that require the expertise of both basic and heavily applied researchers.

Keep in mind that there are also federal Research & Development (R&D) contracts that emphasize the "development" aspects of R&D. Contracts often involve research support for developing designs and prototype components of larger systems, or in some cases the entire system. A large portion of R&D contract support involves missile and aerospace technology, which is very expensive (e.g., NASA, FAA, Navy, Air Force, and Army). From a research career perspective, as a contract PI, you may test hypotheses and publish in scientific journals **unless** a nondisclosure agreement (NDA) is required. Thus, we think it is unlikely that many new academic investigators will see contracted "development work" as career enabling. Table 1.1 summarizes the differences between federal grants and contracts.

Table 1.1 Major differences between federal grants and contracts

Grants	Contracts
Nonbinding – Mechanism to support scientific research to develop new knowledge for the public good	Legally binding – Agreement to acquire goods (e.g., prototypes, computer code, analyses, or services)
Award – Peer review with criteria listed in the Funding Opportunity Announcement	Award – Based on specific evaluation factors listed in the Agency Announcement
Oversight – Government oversight and control is moderate, but not lax – investigator autonomy is usually high	Oversight – Government oversight is moderate to high – investigator autonomy is moderate to low
Deliverables – Final Reports & publications, and occasionally patents	Deliverables – Technical reports, procedures, and/or tangible technology as specified in the contract

1.6.1   Private Sector R&D Contracts

Private sector R&D Contracts differ from public sector research contracts because their focus is more on developing and/or applying prototypes based upon scientific knowledge to technological invention aimed at a marketable product. In addition to aerospace (e.g. Boing, Lockheed), large medical device, pharmaceutical, and service firms continually strive to stay atop of their markets by developing new software systems, compounds, imaging devices, and surgical tools and techniques. This might help to explain why so many tech firms are located on or near university campuses. The cozy proximity facilitates collaboration. Of course, many private sector firms require NDAs just like DOD does. Thus, refereed publications based on private sector contract work must be worked out ahead of time, or researchers risk being denied publication rights. In addition, the contractor likely owns any patents derived from your work, and the contractor's focus is on specific deliverables; not science.

1.6.2   Public/Private Sector Shared R&D Grants

As discussed in Sect. 1.2 above, large universities may seek funding for private sector small business research grants (SBIRs/STTRs), which by intent are used to bring basic research to the marketplace by creating partnerships with industry. Thus, a number of universities have established ties with entrepreneurial businesses. New investigators are unlikely to serve as PIs for small business grants, but you might be invited to work on the project of a senior colleague.

1.6.3   Public Sector R&D Subcontracts

Sometimes university PIs with large federal research grants, subcontract out work to other universities or research institutions because they lack specialized knowledge or technological capabilities. Subcontract money also can be used to support graduate students especially students interested in highly applied research careers. Often grant subcontractors collaborate on scientific research aims and publish jointly, thus in many cases, grant subcontract work is similar to grant research. Nevertheless, contracted research must deliver knowledge and products specified in the contract. These deliverables can include hypothesis testing, software development, measurement tool construction and validation, intervention development and evaluation, and even prototype devices. Depending on the project size and scope, the proposal development process for contracts can be as resource intensive as grant applications. Once you get a federal contract, you are on the hook and committed to the funding agency to deliver very specific products. Use of data for dissertations and publications must be worked out in advance with the contracting institution.

1.7   Cutting Edge Research & Peer Review: The Excitement and the Dilemma

One of the ironies of federally funded research is that "politics" dampens support for cutting edge research. First, in 1976 Congress passed a "*Sense of Congress on Innovation Acceleration Research*" which requires federal agencies to promote cutting-edge research that will break new ground and discover amazing things that will promote the economy, health, and safety of the American people. However, second, Congress want grants to go to institutions in all 435 congressional districts – even ones with no significant research capabilities or staffing. Third, in recent years, some members of Congress (e.g., Senators Proxmire and Coburn) have harshly criticized federal research as not producing anything of value to the American public in order to promote themselves to voters as "watch dogs." (Trager 2015). The inadvertent consequence of conflicting Congressional demands is that the government funds mostly "safe science" – projects likely to find something useful (Catmull 2014). By safe, we mean science that does not take shortcuts, but works incrementally toward understanding. We do not mean valueless science.

To achieve prudent research support in an atmosphere of conflicting political and other demands, agencies have developed impartial peer review systems comprised of top scientists from around the country and elsewhere. When a member of Congress demands to know why their district is not getting its "fair share" of grants, peer review enables agencies to shield themselves with impartial peer reviews. Agencies do try to shelter cutting edge research, that would normally be judged in peer review to be risky by setting aside a relatively small amount of funding for high-risk, high-impact projects. However, such applications receive the highest level of scrutiny during peer review and vetting.

Table 1.2 lists the 7 major review criteria used by NIH and many funding agencies in reviewing applications. The first 5 criteria assess technical merit. Each is assigned an impact score. The last 2 criteria address the projects costs weighed against benefits (contributions as well as harm and other risks) but are not normally considered when assigning a technical merit score. However, the last 2 factors are considered during voting when each reviewer provides an **overall impact score**.

Table 1.2 The major review criteria for NIH grant applications

Technical merit	
1	Significance – The study will produce something that advances science and a recognized public good
2	Investigator(s) – Research will be performed by people with appropriate expertise
3	Innovation – The project is both innovative and based on sound scientific research and theory
4	Approach – The research design will produce a reasonable test of the investigator's hypotheses and will generalize to the target population under study (e.g., gender, race, ethnicity, age groups)
5	Environment – The institution offers adequate resource support
Costs vs. benefits	
6	The public at large as well as human or animal subjects are not at undue risk of harm/discomfort relative to the gain in knowledge. [Unacceptable will disqualify the application for funding.]
7	Costs are reasonable for the budget proposed

Note: Per NIH NOT-OD-17-118, a sixth technical merit criterion applies in the case of clinical trials (discussed later)

Thus, the overall impact score is not necessarily the mean of each reviewer's technical merit scores. Splitting scores like this enables funding institution POs to exercise more flexibility when negotiating budgets or modifying minor human or animal safety procedures. Keep in mind that exercising that flexibility is at the discretion of the funding institution and the PO.

Not only are these 7 criteria applied during peer review, they are also used by everyone in the grant vetting process (Chap. 7). NIH's five major criteria are described in more detail in appendix A. All agencies and foundations have mission-specific and/or award-specific criteria as well (e.g., fellowship training grants differ from research project grants). These are always mentioned in funding opportunity announcements.

In our opinion, the closer a grant application meets the safe-science standard, the higher the likelihood of funding; but the lower the likelihood of cutting-edge research will take place. Why? Because cutting-edge science often fails to pan out empirically. This is in part because such projects take a leap beyond existing findings and/or challenge the utility of generally accepted models and theories.

Before you say to yourself, "Why bother with federal grants if they don't let you explore cutting-edge ideas?" You might consider the following:

- It is probably hubris to assert that your next study will lead to a monumental breakthrough.
- Most studies advance science incrementally rather than creating paradigm shifts.
- A great many novel discoveries occur serendipitously while testing some tangential hypothesis.
- When setting out to do breakthrough science, doing a study to PROVE rather than to FIND OUT, usually raises concerns about investigator bias.

So how can an investigator propose a study with an above-average risk of failure, but that could result in a giant leap forward? We present suggestions later in Chaps. 4 and 5. Before we get to those issues, we want to discuss why you might wish to pursue federal research support (Chap. 2), and what types of support are available (Chap. 3).

References

Catmull, E. (2014). *Creativity, Inc.: Overcoming the unseen forces that stand in the way of true inspiration*. New York: Random House.

Congress. (1976). National science and technology policy, organization, and priorities act of 1976. 42 U.S. Code § 6603 – Sense of Congress on innovation acceleration research. Downloadable from http://uscode.house.gov/view.xhtml?req=(title:42%20section:6603%20edition:prelim).

Finder, A. (2007, November 20). Decline of the tenure track raises concerns. *The New York Times*. Download July 16, 2016 from http://www.nytimes.com/2007/11/20/education/20adjunct.html?module=ArrowsNav&contentCollection=Education&action=keypress&region=FixedLeft&pgtype=article.

Heggeness, M. L., Carter-Johnson, F., Schaffer, W. T., & Rockey, S. J. (2016). Policy implications of aging in the NIH-funded workforce. *Cell Stem Cell, 19*, 15–18.

Jaschik, S. (2009). The disappearing tenure-track job. Inside higher education. Downloaded July 16, 2016 from https://www.insidehighered.com/news/2009/05/12/workforce.

Larson, R. C., Ghaffarzadegan, N., & Xue, Y. (2014). Too many PhD graduates or too few academic job openings: The basic reproductive number R0 in academia. *Systems Research and Behavioral Science, 31*(6), 745–750.

Rockley, S. (2016). What are the chances of getting funded? NIH extramural news. Downloaded July 17, 2016 from https://nexus.od.nih.gov/all/2015/06/29/what-are-the-chances-of-getting-funded/.

Trager, R. (2015). Battle over science funding gets fiercer in U.S. Congress. Scientific American: Chemistry World. Download July 18, 2016 from http://www.scientificamerican.com/article/battle-over-science-funding-gets-fiercer-in-u-s-congress/.

White House Office of Science and Technology Policy (2013). The 2014 Budget: A world-leading commitment to science and research. Washington, DC. Downloaded July 15, 2016 from www.whitehouse.gov/ostp.

GAO (2015). Women in STEM research. Government Accountability Office, Washington, DC

Matthews, K.R.W., Calhoun, K.M., Lo, N., & Ho, V. (2011). The Aging of Biomedical Research in the United States. PLoS ONE 6(12): e29738.

Chapter 2
Pursuing Federal Support

As we mentioned in Chap. 1, free federal money does not mean easy money. **The larger the amount requested, the more detail your application must include, the more scrutiny in review and the more competition your application will face.** Thus, successfully marketing your great ideas requires a lot of thought and strategic, even tactical, planning. That is what grantsmanship is all about.

Without question, the place to start when approaching any agency is to talk to a federal research program official/program director (PO/PD – referred to as a "PO") who knows your field or area of study. At NIH, POs are free to advocate for your project and, time permitting, advise your application development to help you improve its fit with agency needs. This is more common at NIH. Keep in mind that POs are very busy and may administer programs with more than 100 active projects. So, fishing expeditions are unwelcome. It is best to have your questions written out before calling and phrased so as to get a direct clarification or recommended course of action.

Some agencies, like the National Science Foundation (NSF), limit what POs may discuss with applicants because they participate more directly in funding decisions. See Sect. 6.7.2 for more about NSF. At NIH, POs may sit in on reviews (and they do unless there is a conflict or high travel costs), but they are only allowed to observe. Regardless of the agency, emailing a concept paper (See Sect. 4.1) to be followed up with a phone call to see if your great idea might be of interest or mission-appropriate will often get you useful feedback. Your challenge might be to read between the lines in an attempt to detect outright discouragement or a hint of encouragement. In the former case, it might be worthwhile to explore alternative funding institutions.

© The Author(s), under exclusive license to Springer Nature Switzerland AG 2019
T. F. Hilton, C. G. Leukefeld, *Grantsmanship for New Investigators*,
SpringerBriefs in Public Health, https://doi.org/10.1007/978-3-030-01301-1_2

2.1 Myths of Grantsmanship

This section provides our unique perspective of the grants system. We have been on both the applicant and funding sides of the grant and contract process. Over the years, we both have heard so many myths about successful grantsmanship that the metaphor of the blind men and the elephant should be in the minds of all new investigators (older ones too). How and where you interact with the elephant (funding institution) is most likely to generate your working hypothesis of how the system can be favorably influenced.

We've heard absolutely ridiculous ideas even from seasoned PIs with strong grant histories. For example, one academic lab director told Tom that the funding agency program staff were irrelevant to winning a grant. All that was ever necessary to ensure funding was to personally chat with the relevant agency or NIH institute or center (IC) director. That is what they always did, and most of the time they won grants. It just happened that the applications were scientifically solid and highly mission-relevant. The schmoozing was actually annoying. Another senior researcher asserted that agency National Advisory Councils were just a rubber stamp – until a Council rejected one of their favorably reviewed projects. Alas, if an application does not get a meritorious score – it will never get as far as the director for a funding decision. By not engaging with program staff, a PI risks overlooking something that a PO might have readily highlighted as sensitive issue for Council review. The point we want to make here is – be circumspect when listening to advice from colleagues, especially when it does not make logical sense. Most funding institution POs actually do follow the procedures outlined in this book.

The best way to get a handle on agency review processes is to (a) learn how that agency processes applications, (b) identify the kinds of people engaged in reviewing those applications for technical merit (often standing panel member names are publicly available on funding institution websites), and (c) what the review criteria are and how funding decisions are made. A PO can help you understand which panels are best to review your application, and even who is likely to be one or more of the three principle reviewers. Federal FOAs typically contain a lot of information to help ensure that you are informed about the agency mission objectives and any special review criteria. Regardless of available information, many grant applicants either do not take the time to read up on review procedures, or they just can't make sense of the information available. By the time you finish this book, review should make sense. We will discuss grant review more fully in Chap. 6.

Here is a list of some of the most-common grantsmanship myths that we will discuss in this section.

- If I apply, they have to fund me (entitlement)
- I am more likely to get a grant or contract if I pick a hot topic (trending)
- The more work I propose; the better the odds of funding (bargain)
- Ingratiating will increase the odds of getting a grant (schmoozing)
- If I get a good score but am not funded, there is no point in re-applying (petulance)

- Once a grant application is approved, the process is over (i.e., there are no terms and conditions/responsibilities tied to the grant) (naivete)
- As long as I click the submit button at Grants.Gov or HHS ASSIST[1] by the deadline, my application will be reviewed. (what could go wrong?)

2.1.1 If I Apply, They Have to Fund Me

Research grants are not entitlements. You are asking for financial support to conduct research that advances both the nation's scientific knowledge and the mission of a funding organization or agency. Your application goes through several stages of review which are discussed in Chaps. 6 and 7. At each stage, applications are examined using various criteria to gauge suitability for funding. A decision to fund your application might be deferred even if the agency determines that it is solid science and advantageous to it mission. There is only so much money in each agency's or funding institution's budget. In addition, grants are funded in cycles – often quarterly. Thus, your application might be deferred until a future funding cycle. Of course, if the next review cycle identifies highly attractive projects, your grant might keep getting deferred. Periodic checking with your PO will update funding odds. Submitting a revision might be a safer bet.

Even after you are funded, the government can cancel your grant or contract award or reduce it. Cuts and cancellations are most common in DOD, occasional at NSF, but rare at NIH. Asking colleagues who have received support from your target agency regarding the possibility of cuts might influence your budget request. It is always wise to have a fallback plan such as a foundation grant in event of a cut, or the need to scale back the budget to make your project more attractive.

2.1.2 I Am More Likely to Get a Grant or Contract If I Pick a Hot Topic

Some applicants take mission fit so seriously that they think their odds of getting funded improve if the topic is a trending or emerging priority. POs regularly get calls from applicants inquiring; "What's hot?" However, pursuing emergent research topics is usually a risky strategy.

First, pursuing an emergent problem often requires deviating from your established research program. This means that you will be wading into unknown waters – outside your established area of expertise. Your application might not seem to be well-integrated to reviewers. It might contain technical, even fatal flaws. There might even be concerns about the level of expertise presented in the application.

---

[1] You must be registered in Grants.Gov to use the NIH/HHS Application Submission System called ASSIST at https://public.era.nih.gov/assist

Second, it is quite possible that by the time you submit your application, the topic will have been, in Washington DC parlance, **OBE (overcome by events)** and something else has eclipsed it before your scored application has even been vetted for funding.

Finally, there is the case of the federal agency Requests for Applications (RFAs). RFAs often burst onto the scene in response to a perceived epidemic, pending catastrophe, or breakthrough in technology (e.g. CRISPR in genetics). Because RFAs offer a brief window to apply, and a set-aside amount of funds, investigators erroneously see them as less competitive. The idea behind an RFA is that it will attract investigators well positioned to jumpstart the new line of inquiry. However, RFAs increase the risk that a PI will submit an application highly similar to several others with marginally-better scores. The odds of funding for RFAs are roughly the same as unsolicited applications to broad area/program FOAs.

In our opinion, it is always best to work on problems that excite you, have long-standing importance to you and your area of study, and for which you have begun to create a track record of accomplishment as a leader. The odds of submitting an unsolicited application in response to a general FOA that is highly similar to another under review will be relatively low, and you will not have to cope with time and funding constraints circumscribed by an RFA. Tom used to remind grant applicants to pay heed to the Paul Mason motto: "Serve no wine before its time." Carl gave the same message in reference to Michael Angelo's statue of The Thinker. "When it's ready; it's ready."

2.1.3 The More Work I Propose; The Better the Odds of Funding

In product marketing, many companies try to attract buyers by offering more for less. Who doesn't like a bargain, right? The more hypotheses you propose to tests, the more your study might be viewed to be overly complex, analytically challenging, or an over-reach of your expertise. Among successful applicants, 2 or 3 hypotheses are the norm, even for 5-year R01's. We will elaborate on keeping focused throughout the book.

An alternative risk of presenting too many hypotheses or aims is that your application could look like bottom-feeder or catch-all science. Reviewers might conclude that you packed your application with too many aims and/or hypotheses rather than targeting a theoretically important or integrated question. Related to this concern is the potential for reviewers to accuse you of *shotgun empiricism* – Type I error.

Of course, many research designs do allow testing more than 2 or 3 hypotheses, especially with survey research or conducting secondary analyses of large data sets. Keep in mind that the goal of your application is to make a convincing case that investing in your project will advance both science and the funding agency's mission. **You do not need to tell reviewers everything you can or intend to do** as long as the cost of doing so does not exceed the award amount (See also Sect. 6.3).

The limited number of pages in application forms intentionally discourages verbosity. If you and your students publish six or more articles and two dissertations from the study, that's gravy for the funding agency and for your institution. But it is needlessly risky to mention goals that distract reviewers from the primary aims in your application.

Of course, it is possible to err in the opposite direction by presenting too few hypotheses and/or products. Depending on the grant mechanism and budget request, this could risk making your budget appear to be padded. Even if reviewers like your seemingly-bloated application, they may recommend cutting back on an award. Therefore, it's best to present the appropriate science to make the project appear to be worth the financial investment.

2.1.4 Ingratiating Will Increase the Odds of Getting a Grant

Attempting to ingratiate people with influence might advance your interests in some situations, but federal research is not one of them. Research POs are well aware that being a *Golden Goose* draws a lot of attention to them. As POs, we never took flattery and ingratiation seriously. Just be collegial and business-like, and let your relationship with POs in your area of study develop naturally.

Senior PIs (future return customers) sometimes invite all their graduate students and colleagues attending a conference out for dinner and/or drinks. They sometimes invite one or more federal or state agency POs to join the group. This gesture should be carefully considered. To avoid the appearance of a conflict of interest, government employees are generally barred from accepting gifts. Thus, they will insist that they pay their own way. It is okay to invite POs to join your group. Just make sure that you apprise them of the price range on the menu.

Despite these caveats, chatting with POs at meetings and conferences is a reasonable way to test your ideas and help you learn more about the interests of funding institutions. It is not uncommon for POs to offer free professional development workshops (PDWs) as well as conference symposia that describe funding opportunities and interests in addition to explaining their institution's grant vetting process. New investigators especially should attend these PDWs and symposia if they have the opportunity.

2.1.5 If I Get a Good Score but Am Not Funded, There Is No Point in Re-Applying

New investigators seldom win on the first try, and research shows most give up (Heggeness et al. 2016). Given 1-in-4 odds, you should expect to practice your grant-writing skills until you are successful. Many institutions limit resubmissions to one – not NIH. Applicants may resubmit an application to NIH as many times as a PI wishes.

NIH POs will normally encourage PIs to revise and resubmit unless problems raised during review lead them to conclude that it is unlikely to ever be competitive. PIs with a deferred project (scored but not funded) should definitely consider a revise-and-resubmit. If your application is scored but not low enough to expect funding, you have the benefit of the peer review summary statement, which should help you spot your Achilles heels, and eliminate them.

Several weaknesses that are easy to fix include:

- Budget. If your budget is too high and your application has a good score, you could offer to reduce the amount over the phone to see how your PO reacts. He or she might suggest that you eliminate a hypothesis, change the sample size to eliminate a moderator/mediator characteristic, or some other change that will reduce the cost without a commensurate loss in perceived mission value.
- Human/Animal Subjects Protection. A common peer review criticism is insufficient information on procedures for protecting subjects. Review your summary statement and expand your description if human subjects or animal protection issues are identified. Of course, if the concern is not related to omission but rather commission, you might have to revise your design.
- Expertise. Concerns about qualifications are usually aimed at the experience level of the team. A straightforward fix is to include one or two senior colleagues as consultants. Just make sure they have had research grants and are well-published.
- Other Issues. There are many other issues reviewers might raise that often can be fixed or handled within a few weeks without substantially increasing the budget. These can be concerns about analytic approaches, sample size, thoroughness of the literature review, clarity of aims, or measurement tool issues. Once you think you have a fix, call your PO and ask their opinion about your planned changes. Odds are they heard the discussion of your review and can offer deeper insights to expand on what is written on your summary statement.

2.1.6   Once a Grant Application Is Approved, the Process Is Over

Some applicants think that once their application is positively scored, they just need to sit and wait for the money to arrive. However, not all scored applications, even ones with really low scores, are funded. Always check with your PO to get their impression of the likelihood of funding success. Even when your PO shares the encouraging news that you are on the funding plan submitted to their insitution's National Advisory Council, getting an award is not a certainty. Chapter 7 can help to explain why this can be the case in more detail.

In addition, once a project is funded, up, and running; there are "red tape" requirements such as financial reports, progress reports, adverse event reports, and final reports. In between, problems might pop up which require mid-project changes.

Project changes should always be discussed with your PO even if not required by rules or regulations. **Being blind-sided in Washington is the equivalent to Adam and Eve's "Original Sin."** If a problem associated with a discretionary change threatens a delay or requires more funding, you might need financial or other relief to get back on track. Being blindsided by a news headline or Congressional inquiry puts a PO on the spot. It is likely to dampen enthusiasm for bailing you out of a project-related jam.

Finally, **it is a good practice to be working on at least one manuscript for publication every year** of your project – even the first year of a five-year project (See Sect. 2.3.1). Not only is this good for your career, but also it can serve as the material for your grant progress and final reports. Best of all, these publications can be a convincing bridge to your next grant application!

2.1.7 I Only Need to Click the Submit Button at Grants.Gov or ASSIST by the Deadline

A successful application submission means that your institution's federally Authorized Organization Representative (AOR), or perhaps you, have been delegated to transmit an error-free submission to the correct FOA by the deadline. If you click submit, and you receive an error message after the deadline date, then your application will be deferred to the next cycle – even if it is due to a simple administrative flaw, a typo, or a single accidentally-skipped field on a form. We offer more information about application errors to avoid in Sect. 4.3.7.

In addition, before you apply to a federal agency, in fact long before you apply, **you and/or your institution must enroll in Grants.Gov, and for NIH grants, HHS ASSIST.** You, some key team members, and your institution also need to register with NIH[2] and many other target funding agencies. Your *Sponsored Projects* or *Grants Management Offices* should be contacted and must be involved when applying for extramural support. Registrations usually involve providing advanced certifications of your eligibility, such as federal human subjects protection training for key staff or your state vivarium license. Some are mentioned in the federal agency FOA. Others might be on the agency website.

One of the best ways to avoid administrative problems that can disqualify or delay an application review is to get to know your institution's grants office. Finding somebody to coach you on how to avoid snags and technicalities will enhance your success in winning grant awards.

---

[2] https://grants.nih.gov/grants/how-to-apply-application-guide/prepare-to-apply-and-register/register.htm

2.2 Building Your Career One Success at a Time

In academic research, the terms field or area are commonly used to describe a concentration of research in a cluster of related topics focused on making sense and solving problems. The Defense Department, frequently uses the term **"research thrust"** to connote an organized and calculated series of strategic studies that advance toward increased knowledge. Successful research careers can be considered in terms of thrusts as well. Using the thrust metaphor, the more you publish in a particular area; the greater your influence on your peers in that area; the further along that area of science progresses; the more willing agencies will be to fund an evolving and productive line of research; and the quicker you are likely to be thrust into tenure. Alternatively, if your research efforts appear to lack a focused direction, it undermines your ability to exert leadership in your field – in part, this is because you are only contributing data points for other people's meta-analyses.

Science employs an apprenticeship model. Attempts to shortcut that model can result in costly mistakes that risk delaying your research career. In this section, we discuss the three main ways most new investigators build their career using: independent research project grants, postdoctoral grants, and team grants. The independent grants path involves starting with small grants that run a year or less to produce results that justify increasingly longer and larger projects. Postdoctoral career development grants represent a second way to get your research career progressing. This path depends on mentored fellowships and similar research career development grants such as the NIH K awards (Sect. 3.3). A third way is to join an already-funded project team as a co-investigator (Co-I) or consultant. All three paths can be independently pursued or combined based on your unique situation as a scheme for building your research career.

Regardless of the career path chosen, new investigators should adopt the habit of thinking strategically about how the career path(s) they pursue will progressively build their research thrust. By exploring and examining problems in a logical and expanding fashion, you build your reputation as a leading expert in a research area. As your scientific leadership builds, graduate students will be attracted to your lab, and/or research area, and you find yourself coaching their grant applications as you move into the major leagues of academic research.

Moving into the research major leagues is part of grantsmanship. As you build your reputation as a leader in your field, you find yourself being asked to give invited presentations, keynotes, and plenaries. Your reputation at funding agencies eventually will result in being invited to sit on ad hoc advisory committees, and to serve as a permanent study-section reviewer for their grant review programs. Each of these experiences are not only career building, but they also accrue useful experience that gives agencies confidence that your larger projects will be successful for science and the agencies' missions. Aside, it also makes research a very rewarding career choice.

2.2.1 Using Research Project Grants: Starting Small and Building Up

Because science relies on an apprentice model, winning grants is a lot less stressful if you do not get overly ambitious at the start. Both NIH and NSF offer small grants, and because NSF's mission is to promote general science, there is less expectation that an NSF application should meet narrow government needs. The odds are often a bit better when starting out if you apply for less than the maximum amount of funding for a small grant with an eye to building on the success of that first research project grant (RPG). As your program of research, your thrust, grows, you will probably have to shift from NSF to other funding institutions like NIH or large foundations. Because smaller projects often conclude in less than a year, you can compete more often for larger and larger projects until your projects win support for a period of several years.

Applying for grants more frequently has the added advantage of building your application writing and grantsmanship skills. It also requires less paper work, as small grants can have fewer if any progress reporting requirements. As your portfolio builds, it also gives you the flexibility of applying to more than one agency. You might be working on an application to NSF to develop a new analytic procedure, while working on a small 1-year grant from the National Institute on Aging to do secondary data analysis on the role of pain in falls by the elderly, while waiting to hear reviewer reactions to a pending 3-year grant to study the role of pain in prescription drug abuse among the elderly at the National Institute on Drug Abuse.

2.2.2 Using Postdoctoral and Other Career Development Grants

Table 2.1 reflects that NIH and many other federal agencies, have a catalogue of grant mechanisms to support building researcher careers that support their mission. These "career development grants" offer funding mechanisms tailored to help develop new investigators at each stage of their careers. NIH pioneered this type of grant, and therefore offers the most options from high school student to a senior investigator interested in expanding into a new discipline. NSF also supports various research career development grants.

Keep in mind that not all of these grants are available to everyone, all the time. Some are issued only when research is justified by scientific need. Some of these grants are limited to US citizens or US residents, whereas others are only available to applicants who are not US citizens. Similarly, some grants are only available to pre-doctoral students while others are only available to post-doctoral students. Some are only available to clinicians whereas others are only available to seasoned researchers. Several career development grants are focused on minorities, or underfunded institutions.

Table 2.1 Examples of federal grants available to support the development of new researchers

PRE-DOC
Institutional (in-house) training
Undergraduate training
Graduate training
Dissertation support
POST-DOC
Postdoctoral fellowship
Career transition from clinician to scientists
Pathway to research independence

2.2.3 Starting in the Trenches: Joining Somebody Else's Grant

Another way to start out is to join an already-funded project as a Co-I, research associate, consultant, statistician, or some other role. Ideally, finding a team with a funded project in your own university or department is ideal. Although it is best to find a project in your immediate vicinity, it is not essential. However, because distance will insulate you from the daily turmoil of working on a grant – you're less likely to learn useful project management skills if you are not near the team geographically.

Once you have been on a project for a year or so, you might ask the PI to help you submit a supplemental grant that enables you to pursue independent interests. Yes, there are supplemental grants. Although supplements are most often used by agencies to ensure a grant succeeds in the event of catastrophe, supplements are small projects that spin off existing project grants in order to pursue hypotheses emanating from the larger project. An example might be to explore an unforeseen mediator or moderator effect. Another might be to examine a hypothesis from a novel perspective such as the role of messenger RNA in a neuroscience study.

Even if you get a supplement grant, you still have to be focused on getting an RPG as PI. We have known researchers who have held Co-I status on various grants for a decade or more before striking out as PI for the first time. Some scientific areas require longer apprenticeships than others, in part because the technology can be highly complex. Working as a Co-I can provide valuable experience in managing large projects requiring a project team to conduct. It also can enable you to spend more time publishing. However, your support rests on the success of the senior PI, and that is not a guarantee.

How can you discover colleagues in your area who are working on projects for which the PI might welcome your participation as an asset? RePorter (projectre-porter.nih.gov) enables complex searchers of all NIH funded projects that includes institution and geographic location. NSF has a similar database called Research. gov. Tom has used the RePorter database to help new or recently-relocated investigators identify nearby expertise to flesh out their teams as well as help new investigators identify PIs who might be interested in working with them.

2.3   Publish or Perish

You get to become a leader in your field one publication at a time. Even though many academics disdain the phrase, the bromide "publish or perish" is a truism when it comes to leadership in science. Faculty who get early tenure and promotions are those who publish more total articles, publish more articles in top-tier journals, sit on editorial boards, serve on federal peer review panels, and eventually become journal editors (Fairweather 2005; Hong and Honig 2016; O'Keefe and Wang 2013). So, as publications build, that history offers evidence to reviewers that your next project will be a success.

2.3.1   How to Start Publishing the First Year

A strategy we have observed among the most successful grantees is that they try to publish at least one paper each award year plus one other publication. Thus, a three-year grant should produce four papers. But – how can you write a paper on a project when you have only begun to collect the data? In many cases, applicants have done much of the library work that could be used to write a review paper building on the literature cited in their application. Perhaps you developed new measures, unique statistical or other procedures that can be published. Perhaps you used a unique recruiting method that resulted in high enrollment. One of Toms' grantees published a paper (Scott 2004) on retention of subjects for long-range follow-ups that is today a citation classic! These are all topics that do not always need to wait for final results.

Even though mid-project your database is still growing, you might have completed a validation of your assay methods or survey measures. Sometimes projects encounter unforeseen barriers that had to be overcome. How you overcame that barrier might be of interest to colleagues. These are examples of how to possibly publish every year of a project. We say "plus one" because after the final results are in, depending on how hypothesis testing turned out, there is usually one or more papers to write up the final results.

2.3.2   What If My Hypotheses Are Not Supported by the Data?

What if your study fails to refute the null hypothesis? Who will publish those results? Is it a MYTH that journals will not publish negative findings? Think about effect sizes for example. If all effect sizes were the same, there would be no meta-analyses. John Ioannidis at Stanford is a perfect example of a researcher who has made a successful career challenging non-replicable healthcare studies. This suggests that there is gold even in what appears to be a played-out data mine. However, the trick is to describe a class half-full; not half-empty.

For a great many researchers, identify publishable issues highlighted by failure to support hypotheses is a challenge. However, articles that fail to replicate prior studies are increasingly being published. Many of these publications discuss implications for design, analyses, and/or theory. Therefore, unexpected research results can help to inform science about issues that can improve future research. Strategically, a lot seems to rest with the title – a glass half-full or half-empty. "Failure to replicate the XYZ theory in the study of ABC" might get a superficial review. Alternatively, "When the XYZ theory fails to predict: Implications for the study of ABC" is a title more likely to receive attention. If the manuscript presents flawed prior assumptions, identifies analytic issues, and/or includes a constructive modification of the theory or approach, all the better.

Finally, if your research failed to replicate a published study as expected, that could become a segue to a follow-on grant to explore alternative methods, applications, statistics, or sampling depending upon how results are characterized. It might be that the theory only needs refinement.

References

Fairweather, J. (2005). Beyond the rhetoric: Trends in the relative value of teaching and research in faculty salaries. *The Journal of Higher Education, 76*, 401–422.

Heggeness, M. L., Carter-Johnson, F., Schaffer, W. T., & Rockey, S. J. (2016). Policy implications of aging in the NIH-funded workforce. *Cell Stem Cell, 19*, 15–18.

Hong, Y., & Honig, B. (2016). Publish and politics: An examination of business school faculty salaries in Ontario. *Academy of Management Learning & Education, 15*(4), 665–685.

O'Keefe, S., & Wang, T. C. (2013). Publishing pays: Economists' salaries reflect productivity. *The Social Science Journal, 50*, 45–54.

Scott, C. K. (2004). A replicable model for achieving over 90% follow-up rates in longitudinal studies of substance abusers. *Drug and Alcohol Dependence, 74*(2004), 21–36.

Chapter 3
Grant Mechanisms

As previously mentioned, Federal agencies offer a myriad of grant mechanisms as a way to invest in science and scientists. Each agency has developed their own programs and structures which can be perused on Grants.Gov, creating a veritable alphabet soup of grant mechanism designators, shorthand's for different types of grants. Shorthand designations like K23 or P30 are always spelled out and operationally defined in FOAs. Each mechanism delineates a maximum award amount and time period, special qualifications for applicants, submission deadlines, the purpose of the grant mechanism, mission aims, and any special review criteria.

Our focus here is to overview the six general categories of grant mechanisms.

- Research project grants (RPGs),
- Training grants,
- Career development grants,
- Application/implementation grants,
- Conference grants
- Project planning grants

Most US grant opportunities are not available to foreign institutions unless there is an obvious payoff to the US.

3.1 Research Project Grants (RPGs)

Research project grants (RPGs) are the backbone of NIH and NSF federal research grant portfolios. They are awarded to universities and research institutions to conduct studies aimed at advancing the public interest of the United States. These grants may also be studies that advance space exploration, reduce crime, improve the public health, or protect the nation from its enemies. Generally, RPGs come in small medium, large, and extra-large sizes. They may be unsolicited and based on FOAs called Program Announcements or Broad Area Announcements (PA/BAA) or

© The Author(s), under exclusive license to Springer Nature Switzerland AG 2019
T. F. Hilton, C. G. Leukefeld, *Grantsmanship for New Investigators*,
SpringerBriefs in Public Health, https://doi.org/10.1007/978-3-030-01301-1_3

solicited Request for Applications/Proposals (RFA/RFP) to meet emergent needs. Normally, new investigators will be applying for small and medium-sized grants using PA or BAA FOAs.

Small Grants NIH and NSF award most small Federal grants. Normally, small grants have a funding ceiling of under $250 K and are completed in 2 years or less. The NIH R03 is a good example. **R03s are perhaps the most popular grant mechanism to help PIs at any career stage to justify a subsequent R01 or other large-budget grant application.** R03s are rarely renewable. R03 grants are for up to 2 years with a direct cost limit of $50 K/year. They most often support pilot or feasibility studies, collection of preliminary data; secondary analysis of existing data; small, self-contained research projects; or development of new research technology.

Although not considered a small grant, PIs may submit small R01s. The R01 should be used only if the project must be longer than 2 years and/or the total direct costs will exceed $100 K. Although uncommon, it is acceptable for an R01 that asks for $30 K/year for 3 or 4 years if the design warrants it. One caveat about small R01s is that if you are a new or early-stage investigator (NI/ESI), you might lose your status at NIH – check with an NIH PO.

Medium-Sized Grants Medium sized grants are the mainstay of university research. They usually have a total ceiling of about $2.5 M, are renewable (competitively), and must be completed within 5 years or less. The NIH R01 is typical. These grants form the fundamental building blocks of new theories and new discoveries. They are large enough to produce generalizable results, yet small enough to make subsequent replication studies affordable. By providing focused studies, medium-sized grants are the grist of meta-analyses used to cross-validate theories and empirical discoveries. Needless to say, most science is carried out with medium-sized grants. There is no specific dollar limit unless specified in the FOA, however, advance permission is required for an amount over $500 K in any single year of the grant.

R15 is a special type of medium-sized grant called the Academic Research Enhancement Award (AREA). They are earmarked for universities receiving less than $6 M/year in total federal grant support, and they require significant student involvement. These are 3-year research grants and are capped at $300 K in direct costs. Historically, R15 grants have been limited in number.

R21 is NIH's Exploratory/Developmental Research Grant Award (R21). We like this mechanism as it offers more support than an R03 for pilot and feasibility studies. Like R03s, R21s run for 2 years, but their budget maxes out at $275 K vs $100 K.

Large Grants Large RPGs can support institutionally-based research centers (P01s), modest-sized cooperative projects involving multiple institutions (U01s), or just one big, expensive project in a single R01 RPG. Large grants normally lack a defined budget ceiling, but often require permission to submit. The time commitment is usually for 5–10 years before a competitive renewal application is required. Large grants are intended to sustain a complex infrastructure and technology needed to study high-priority problems. They can be used to create or expand centers of excellence that attract a number of experts to a single organization for improved collaboration. Usually, award parameters for large grants are specified in the FOA. For example, "The agency has set aside up to $40 M to support up to 8 institutions for up to 5 years with a possibility of renewal for up to 5 additional years."

Extra-Large Grants These RPGs (UM1/2) are rare and only periodically announced. They are often multi-institution and/or multi-center, involve a dozen or more research institutions, and the cost can exceed a billion dollars over the life of the project. The NIH Human Genome Project is an example. Most extra-large projects extend more than 8 years, are sometimes renewable (i.e. re-competed), and usually cost between $30 M and $250 M for the whole project across all participating grantee institutions.

3.2   Training Grants

Training grants range from supporting high school curricula to funding postgraduate study. Training grants fall into two categories: T (training) and F (fellowship) grants. T-grants are unique among career development grants since they are awarded to educational institutions. Grantees are responsible for curriculum development, instruction, and deciding on student eligibility for stipends and other financial support. The NIH T32 is a typical training grant. It covers tuition, fees, and stipends to support students in a training program as well as conference travel, lab equipment, and faculty salaries.

Training grants also may include cross training to enable interdisciplinary research, career transitions from clinician to researcher, and to help people sidelined by illness or other life events to obtain refresher training to re-enter their field. Table 3.1 summarizes the types of training grants supported by NIH.

Fellowship grants are usually awarded to individuals, either directly by the funding institution or indirectly by an educational institution. Fellowships include both pre- and postdoctoral study at virtually any career stage. Most common are fellowship grants to support pre-doctoral student dissertation research or to extend mentored research following the award of a doctorate. Some fellowship grants are open to foreign applicants to study in the US.

If a pre-doctoral researcher knows what he or she needs and where they are going career-wise, there is likely to be a grant mechanism to help get there and even go beyond their post-doctoral career. We suggest that you always discuss applying for a grant with your academic advisor and/or your major professor. If you are still undecided, do not be bashful about talking to fellow students who have one of these types of grants, and talk to other trusted faculty and friends. Our experience suggests

Table 3.1 Types of training grants

T32	**Ruth L. Kirschstein Institutional National Research Service Award** enables institutions to recruit individuals selected by the program leadership for pre-doctoral and/or postdoctoral research training in specified scientific areas
T34	**Ruth L. Kirschstein Undergraduate NRSA Institutional Research Training Grants** enhance the undergraduate research training of individuals from groups underrepresented in biomedical and behavioral sciences through Institutional NRSA training grants, in preparation for research
T35	**Ruth L. Kirschstein NRSA Short-Term Institutional Research Training Grant** provide individuals with research training during off-quarters or summer periods to encourage research careers and/or research in areas of national need
T/ R90	**Ruth L. Kirschstein Interdisciplinary Research Training Award (T90) and combined Research Education Grant (R90)** support comprehensive interdisciplinary research training programs at the undergraduate, predoctoral and/or postdoctoral levels, by capitalizing on the infrastructure of existing multidisciplinary and interdisciplinary research programs
T15	**Continuing Education Training Grants** assist professional schools to establish, expand, or improve programs of continuing professional education, or refresher education dealing with new developments in the science of technology of the profession. [Availability follows national needs and may not be available in some years
D43	**International Research Training Grants** support research training programs for U.S. and foreign professionals and students to strengthen global health research and international research collaboration
D71	**International Research Training Planning Grants** enable planning for the preparation of an application for a D43 international research training grant or for a U2R international research training cooperative agreement

that applications which reflect a clear vision and a reasoned path to achieve career goals have the best success. Keep in mind that career development grants are not entitlements, and there are many of your peers who are also applying at the same time.

Many fellowship grants (F awards) pay tuition and fees. Some include a modest stipend to pay for living expenses. Most F awards are limited to US citizens or permanent residents. Table 3.2 describes grant mechanisms to support the educational development of students pursuing research careers.

3.3   Career Development Awards

Career Development Awards (CDAs; or K grants; see Table 3.3) rely upon diverse mechanisms because individual careers tend to be unique. K grants can range from mentored postdoctoral training to special support for leaders in a research area. The NIH K01 is a typical career development award, and not unlike some T grants, they involve one or more mentors. Awardees must be full-time affiliates of the applying institution and be US citizens, nationals of a US possession or territory (e.g., Samoa) or be permanent US residents at the time of award. There is some overlap between

Table 3.2 Types of fellowship grants

F05	**International Research Fellowships** provide collaborative research opportunities for qualified foreign scientists who hold a doctoral degree or its equivalent in the biomedical or behavioral sciences. [availability follows national needs and may not be available in some years.]
F30	**Ruth L. Kirschstein Individual Predoctoral NRSA for MD/PhD and other Dual Degree Fellowships** support pre-doctoral training aimed at dual Clinical/Research degrees such as the MD/PhD
F31	**Ruth L. Kirschstein Predoctoral Individual National Research Service Awards** provide pre-doctoral individuals with supervised research training in specified health and health-related areas leading toward the research doctoral degree (e.g., PhD)
F32	**Ruth L. Kirschstein Postdoctoral Individual National Research Service Awards** provide postdoctoral research training to individuals to broaden their scientific background and extend their potential for research in specified health-related areas
F33	**Ruth L. Kirschstein National Research Service Awards for Senior Fellows** provide opportunities for experienced scientists to make major changes in the direction of research careers, or to acquire new research capabilities to engage in health-related research
F99/ K00	**Individual Predoctoral to Postdoctoral Fellow Transition Awards** support Pre- to Post-doctoral transition of highly motivated graduate students. The F99 activity code is intended to only be used in conjunction with a K00 Award. [Availability follows national needs and may not be available in some years.]

NIH T and K grants, so if you are contemplating a career development grant, make sure to check both mechanisms.

The most hybrid of the K's is the NIH Pathway to Independence (PI) Award (K99/R00). Sometimes called Kangaroo grants, K99/R00 grants are intended to help postdocs who are no more than 4 years out of school to leap from a mentored situation into tenure-track research independence. The grant devotes the first part to a mentored phase (1–2 years) that will prepare the new researcher to execute an R00 research project (2–3 years) if they have landed a tenure-track position. Basically, Kangaroos offer a university or research institution a cost-free "tryout." They hire NIs/ESIs on the government's grant money to see if you can support yourself before committing to a permanent position.

3.4 Application/Implementation Grants (Small Business Grants)

The Small Business Innovative Research Grant (SBIR) and its sibling, the Science Technology Transfer Grant (STTR), are the most prominent among funding mechanisms that help to transition science into application. The difference between the two is somewhat vague. The main difference lies in whether or not the PI is an academic researcher (STTR) or a small business owner who teams up with an academic researcher (SBIR). The US Small Business Administration requires that all

Table 3.3 Types of K career development grants

K01	**Mentored Research Scientist Career Development Awards** support postdoctoral or early career research scientists committed to research, in need of both advanced research training and additional experience
K02	**Independent Research Scientist Development Awards** support early to mid-career scientists with research funding who need of additional protected time (usually from a teaching load) for research activities
K05	**Senior Research Scientist Awards** support senior researchers with research funding to pursue independent research and to serve as a mentor to more junior research scientists
K07	**Academic Career Development Awards** support either a mentored or independent investigator to develop or enhance curricula, foster academic career development of promising young teacher-investigators, and to strengthen existing teaching programs
K08	**Mentored Clinical Scientist Research Career Development Awards** support promising clinician-scientists with demonstrated aptitude to develop into independent investigators, or for faculty members to pursue research, and aid in filling the academic faculty gap in health profession's institutions
K12	**Clinical Scientist Institutional Career Development Program Awards** support newly-trained clinicians appointed by an institution for development of independent research skills and experience in a fundamental science within the framework of an interdisciplinary research and development program
K18	**Research Career Enhancement Award for Established Investigators** provides either full-time or part-time support to broaden individual research capabilities or to make changes in one's research career by acquiring new research skills or knowledge
K22	**Career Transition Awards** support outstanding newly-trained basic or clinical investigators to develop their independent research skills through a two-phase program; an initial mentored research experience, followed by a period of independent research (see also K99/R00)
K23	**Mentored Patient-Oriented Research Career Development Awards** support the career development of clinically-trained professionals who have made a commitment to patient-oriented research, and who have the potential to develop into productive, clinical investigators
K24	**Midcareer Investigator Award in Patient-Oriented Research** support mid-career clinicians with research support who need protected time to devote to patient-oriented research and to serve as mentors for beginning clinical investigators
K25	**Mentored Quantitative Research Career Development Awards** support investigators with quantitative scientific and engineering backgrounds outside of biology or medicine who have made a commitment to focus their research endeavors on basic or clinical biomedical research
K26	**Midcareer Investigator Awards** in Biomedical and Behavioral Research support biomedical and behavioral scientists who need protected time to devote to their research and mentoring
K43	**Emerging Global Leader Awards** support research and provides protected time to international junior scientists with a faculty positions in low to middle-income countries leading to an independently funded research career
K76	**Emerging Leaders Career Development Awards** support the development of US resident physician-scientists prepared to take an active role in leading transformative change on a global level in biomedical research enterprise
K99/	**Pathway to Independence Awards** support an initial mentored research experience (K99)

(continued)

Table 3.3 (continued)

R00	followed by independent research (R00) for highly qualified, postdoctoral researchers, to secure an independent research position. Award recipients are expected to compete successfully for independent R01 support during the R00 phase

federal agencies provide SBIR and STTR grants. Regardless of the role of the PI, both researchers and business developers must be involved. However, there are limits to the amount of funds available, and usually these grants are not renewable. Application/Implementation grants can be used by academic researchers to start a small business in order to profit from their findings, or to help a business partner develop a joint venture. For example, Tom encouraged several SBIR grants to help add new modules to commercial statistical packages in order to increase researcher access to new analytic tools. Similarly, some of the SBIR grants in his portfolio supported making addiction recovery smartphone apps and expanding existing commercially-available medical screening and diagnostic batteries.

R43/R44 is NIH's version of the SBIR, and the R41/R42 supports STTRs. Both R43 and R41 grants support 6–12 months to establish the scientific and technical merit of the proposal (usually capped at $150 K). If the PI can make the case that research to commercialize is justified, there is usually an additional 2-year R44 or R42 grant award of up to $500 K/year. Applicants must be US small businesses to meet SBA criteria. Can you request more than the cap amount? Yes, but you usually must get permission from the funding agency to submit an application with a higher cost or it will not be reviewed.

3.5 Conference Grants

Did you ever wonder about the origin of scientific conferences you never heard of before? Well, if some federal agencies see a useful learning opportunity, they can help fund conferences. One of the most common reasons to fund a conference is to enhance peer-to-peer communication, especially in an emerging field or a field that has a high priority to their mission. The HIV epidemic offered a sound rationale for stimulating trans-disciplinary, international collaboration. Sometimes, one can sell a conference idea as being a stimulus for interest in an important research area in which research activity has been declining. The NIH R13 is a typical conference grant mechanism. How much can you request? That varies with the funding institution budget, and how good you are at negotiating. Like many grants, it is good if you can recruit interested co-sponsors to spread the cost. Some R13s are initiated when a conference committee needs to augment its funds or risk meeting cancellation.

3.6 Planning Grants

Yes, you can get funded to see if you want to apply for grant support, or to gather information to justify support. So-called planning grants are sometimes necessary to explore the best structure for a complex project that might involve multiple institutions, federal agencies, and/or diverse specialties. The NIH R34 is an example. These grants are often used to set up cooperative research projects and large clinical trials (See Sect. 5.4.2). Basically, R34s are designed to avoid the *"Field of Dreams"* type of risk (named after the movie). Instead of assuming that if you build it they will come, it supports answering such questions as: "If we build it, will they come?" and "Can we build it at all?" or "If we try to build it, can we assemble the right team and materials?" Institutions considering creating a research center or a large training grant program can apply for a planning grant. It is common for NIH POs to invite such applications when considering a large grant initiative. These grants often build momentum at meetings and conferences where diverse interests are converging on a research need.

Chapter 4
The Application Process

This chapter is intended to help you think strategically when drafting an application by helping you better understand how agencies actually arrive at final funding decisions. The process depicted in Fig. 4.1 can be circuitous at various stages, but it is rational – even commonsensical. Your strategic plan should be focused on convincing peer reviewers and funding agency/institution staff that **your research question is solid**, **your hypotheses are worthy of testing**, and **the manner in which you propose to test them is sound**. To develop your strategic plan, you need to have a roadmap to help identify where obstacles are likely to present themselves at each stage of the application process. Most funding institutions follow a roadmap similar to that for NIH in Fig. 4.1. Hopefully, as you proceed through each step of the application process, you will develop tactics to either overcome or avoid barriers altogether until you reach your ultimate strategic objective – a grant.

Figure 4.1 depicts the dynamics of the typical life cycle of an NIH grant. You start with an idea for a project, get feedback from various sources, sketch out a plan to explore the project's feasibility, and enlist human and other resources needed for the project. You then draft your research plan in accordance with required rules and forms, submit it for review, revise and resubmit your plan if it does not review well, otherwise wait to hear if it is fundable. If your project is considered for funding, you negotiate any final issues, get your grant award, and start the study.

Post-award, you still have to keep your funding institution informed about progress, and deal with any problems that arise during the project, while publishing journal articles along the way. Toward the end of the project, you have to determine if you want to pursue new hypotheses related to the problem by competing to continue a new phase of the project, or to start something new. In either case, the cycle starts all over again. Chap. 5 will discuss content issues, Chap. 6 will overview the application review process, and Chap. 7 will address the final phase of pursuing a grant; vetting fundable projects, award decisions, and ultimately, applying for funding to address your next project.

© The Author(s), under exclusive license to Springer Nature Switzerland AG 2019   37
T. F. Hilton, C. G. Leukefeld, *Grantsmanship for New Investigators*,
SpringerBriefs in Public Health, https://doi.org/10.1007/978-3-030-01301-1_4

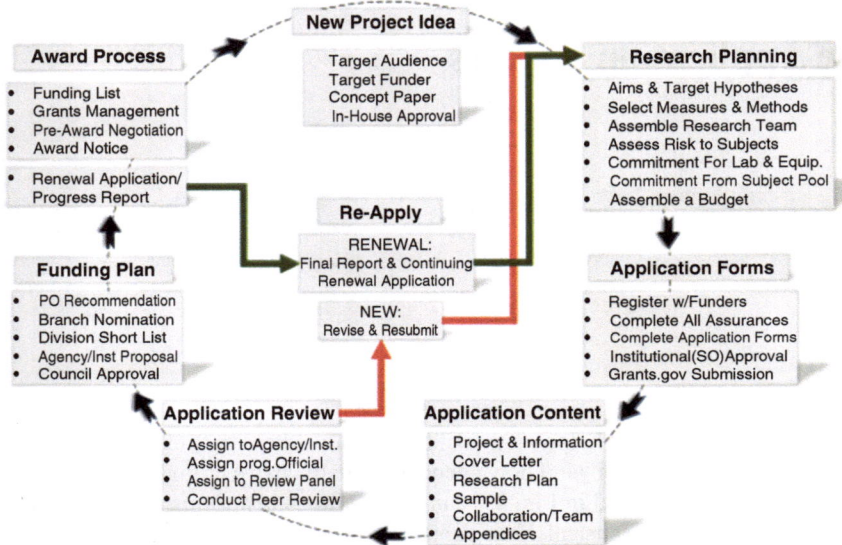

Fig. 4.1 A graphic depiction of the life cycle of a research grant

Figure 4.1 may seem overwhelming. It is not much different from your dissertation process. It also underscores that there is a lot of collaboration along the way. Your university or research institution has staff members familiar with the grant application rules and procedures of most agencies and many other funding institutions to help you navigate the formal application process. **We strongly suggest that you visit your institution's grants management / sponsored research office, and engage their help**, even if your department or school does not require it. Your job as investigator is to present a credible case for funding your project. Their job is to help you meet all the bureaucratic requirements to comply with applicable rules, regulations, and forms.

The remaining sections of this book will follow the roadmap diagram presented in Fig. 4.1 one stage at a time, and discuss what is involved, what obstacles you should be prepared to address, and even offer a tip now and then on strategies for overcoming the more commonly-experienced ones.

4.1 Project Idea

New Project Idea

- Target Audience
- Target Funder
- Concept Paper
- In-House Approval

Your project idea, and the research question upon which your project will focus, is the first step in the application process. You will need to flesh out your idea and define the parameters and the focus of your study so that you can briefly articulate your concept to others. Normally, you will start with your mentor, then colleagues, your department chair, and whomever else whose knowledge and experience you can rely upon as you start the application process.

4.1.1   Target Audience & Targeted Funding Institution

One of the most rewarding, if not fun, parts of science is coming up with new ways to examine the world and improve our understanding of it. Sometimes ideas and research questions come as hunches out of the blue, but most of the time, they come from observations in our own labs/settings or from reading the reports of colleagues. When moving from an idea and key questions to a planned-out project, the first thing to consider is your audience. The audience is the group who will most benefit from your research. Identifying your target audience helps you narrow the focus of your project aims and literature review. It also suggests which funding institution(s) has a large enough stake in your project's outcomes that they might be motivated to pay for it.

4.1.2   Concept Paper

Before you talk to anybody aside from your immediate mentor or colleagues about your idea, you should draft a concept paper. Table 4.1 lists the essential information for a concept paper.

The Table 4.1 topics are also key topics that must be addressed in your formal application, so you can think of your concept paper as the outline of your application. The process of writing your idea down on paper (docx & pdf) will help organize (and revise) your thoughts, and the thoughts of those whom you need to convince as your application progresses. Start by assembling a brief 1–4-page description of your project. You might revise it over time as your planning narrows your focus and enables greater specificity. Your concept paper will also be key to engaging interest and support from superiors, colleagues, and often staff at your target funding institution before you commit more time and resources to pursuing a grant or contract. Your concept paper will also come in handy later in the process to help recruit members of your research team as well as lining up sources for access to research subjects, lab space, equipment, and other resources.

Table 4.1 Essential elements of a 1 to 6-page research project concept paper

1. Purpose/aims and **question:** What is the purpose or main aims of your project and the research question? Will it examine a theory/model to guide which hypotheses you test?
2. Significance: What is the payoff to science, the funding institution's mission, and the public?
3. Problem/background: Why you to think this topic needs study? – What's in it for science and the public?
(a) Clinical/scientific relevance
(b) Gap in knowledge
(c) Fit with long-term program of your lab
(d) Theoretical & practical objective of this study
4. Design: What is the design that will enable testing your hypotheses? Sample, intervention, controls, measures, etc.
5. Analysis: What is your statistical approach & analysis plan? Why is it optimal?
6. Innovation: How and why is the project innovative?
7. Team: Who will be doing the work and what are their qualifications / experience?
8. Logistics: Do you have population access? Do you have access to necessary equipment and lab space? What is the **level of effort** to be invested (see Sect. 4.3.1): staffing required, study duration, and cost?

4.1.3   In-House Approval

Armed with a clear and convincing concept paper, you are ready to approach others in your institution for comment. The "idea stage" of the application process varies from institution to institution, but it usually begins by chatting with your mentor or department head, and possibly meeting with your institution's Authorized Organization Representative (AOR) aka "Signing Official." The AOR may be a chair, dean or other administrative official who has the authority to commit resources and sign agreements on behalf of your university or research institution. The AOR acts as a gatekeeper and ensures that research is done "by the book." This includes accepting responsibility to ensure all research activity conforms to all applicable laws, rules, and regulations. It is the AOR who communicates with the funding institution for your institution, because **normally, your institution is the grant awardee – not you.**

4.2   Research Planning

Research Planning

- Aims & Target Hypotheses
- Select Measures & Methods
- Assemble Research Team
- Assess Risk to Subjects
- Commitment For Lab & Equip.
- Commitment From Subject Pool
- Assemble a Budget

Before you can assemble a grant application, thorough planning is critical. After the purpose and research question, foremost is deciding on the specific aims of your project and the hypotheses you intend to focus on. Getting this right will really help you succeed in getting funded. Without good science, nothing else is likely to make your grant application or contract proposal competitive. However, to make it a good investment, requires **minimizing apparent risk.** Peer reviewers judge both the scientific merit of your project and its viability. The greater the likelihood that the project will not produce new knowledge, or fail to produce anything at all, the riskier the project will appear. There is also risk associated with perceptions of how well your project will advance the funding institution's mission and promote some public good relative to competing projects. Everyone in the vetting process seeks to determine a research project grant's investment risk. Therefore, the weight placed on each criterion at each stage of the review and vetting process in Fig. 4.1, influences reviewers' overall impressions of the following risks:

1. <u>Applicant Resources</u>. Is the applicant's university or research institution providing appropriate resources such as manpower, talent, equipment, subject access, and subject protection to achieve the aims?
2. <u>Applicant Expertise</u>. Do the PI and other key members of the research team have the training and expertise to successfully lead and conduct the proposed project?
3. <u>Soundness</u>. Is the proposed project based on sound logic and empirical principles justified by the existing research findings in the literature?
4. <u>Study Aims</u>. Is the proposed project well-aligned with the funding institution's mission, administration, and congressional priorities (if appropriate)?
5. <u>Urgency</u>. Are the timing, the costs, and other resources appropriate to advance the funding institution's mission - usually public health, welfare, or safety?

One possible way to help you think strategically about a grant application is to think about it like applying for a car loan. Suppose you are a single postdoc applying for a $30,000 car loan for a new Honda Civic. At the same time a tenured professor in your department applies for the same loan on an identical car. Strategically, you both want to convince your funding institution, the bank, that you will not default on their investment in you, and thus further their mission of issuing profitable car loans.

The bank turns down your loan application, because of your low stipend and little or no credit history. The professor is offered a 5% APR loan because she has a good credit history although she has a mortgage and an outstanding loan on a washer and dryer. You need a car, so you decide to ask for a $10,000 loan on a used Honda Civic. From the bank's perspective, that request better aligns with your capacity to repay the loan reducing the risk of their investment. The bank offers you a loan at 5.4% APR.

You both try to negotiate better loan terms. The professor decides to make a $7000 down payment from her saving account. That lowers her loan to $23,000 and the bank lowers her APR to 4.2%. You try to lower the risk associated with your loan by getting your father to co-sign your loan. The bank, in turn, lowers your rate to

4.9%. Both of you selected more achievable **goals** (lower loan amounts). Your dad's cosigning indicated a good-faith effort to reassure the bank that it will get **reliable** payments. Both applications lowered the perceived **risk** of failure to repay and you both got the car. This hypothetical story is a metaphor for a revise-and-resubmit grant application.

Thinking strategically, as an early-stage researcher, includes three tactics you can pursue to minimize the apparent risk of your application:

(a) GOAL: Ask for enough support to meet all requirements to achieve aims – BUT don't appear to be overreaching (that used Honda vs a new one).
(b) RELIABILITY: Include experienced collaborators with a history of success upon whom you can rely – Co-Is.
(c) RISK: Describe potential barriers to success and identify resources sufficient to overcome them in event they occur – consultants and assistants (like cosigner dad).

4.2.1 Aims and Target Hypotheses

Your aims, what you want to accomplish, set the tone for your application. Logically, they should not only be clear in your mind, but easily articulated when writing and talking about them with others. Normally your hypotheses follow from your research aims. So, logically, **the number of aims, like the number of hypotheses, should rarely exceed three** for an R01. Extra-Large grants like Center Grants or large Cooperatives might have one or two additional aims.

One of the reasons we recommend making your case using one to three aims and hypotheses is that it becomes increasingly difficult for the human brain to track more than 3 things at once. Thus, adding aims and hypotheses increases the odds of confusion for the reviewers. It also risks giving reviewers the impression that you are over-reaching or that your thinking has not fully matured and that the project might wander in unproductive directions. We will discuss hypotheses further in Sect. 4.3.4.

Can you test more than 3 hypotheses? Nearly always! And, you should have plans to do that whenever possible. However, page limitations constrain what you can tell reviewers you intend to do. Trying to tell them everything you hope to achieve will inevitably result in critical omissions. For example, your literature review will likely seem inadequate, methodological details will be too sparse, how you intend to analyze your data may seem confusing, etc. You want to provide enough information to ensure that both peer reviewers and the funding institution will view your project to be great science and worthy of their support. Put differently, **present enough information to justify a grant award – not everything you plan to do when you get the grant**. If you and your students publish six or more articles and two dissertations from the study, that's gravy for the funding agency and for your institution. But it is needlessly risky to mention goals unrelated to the primary aims in your application.

4.2.2   Selection of Measures & Methods

Your application must present sound methodology and measurement techniques. Since your competitiveness often hinges on innovative methods and approaches to measurement, precision is critical here. For example, you want to present a clear description of the design including what and how biological, behavioral, and/or lab measures will be used. This is the section to incorporate previous and commonly-used study designs and validated measures, including validity and reliability citations for each instrument. Statistical approaches to test each hypothesis should be specifically described, and if necessary justified. If human subjects are involved, for example, a power analysis must be presented to ensure an adequate sample size. We strongly recommend involving a person with statistical and measurement expertise from application phase through to the final reports unless that expert is you.

4.2.3   Assembling a Research Team

Science is a team endeavor. Think about what skills are needed to successfully complete the study as well as including established scientists, research assistants, Co-Is and/or consultants to help avoid pitfalls. Doing so lowers perceived risk by reviewers.

Everybody is busy, so getting colleagues to get on board with your possibly-maybe-hopefully-to-be-funded project means not taking too big a chunk out of their busy schedules in the event that you get the grant. Yours may not be the only project in the wings to which they have signed on. Colleagues who are very enthusiastic about your project may wish to be involved at half or even full time. Just keep in mind that if you bring on high-profile Co-Is or consultants at very low percentages of time, they not only look like window-dressing; they ARE window dressing. This will undermine reassuring reviewers that people have your back if you get into a jam. On the other hand, the more time on the project, the higher will be its cost.

4.2.4   Assessing Risks to Human and Animal Subjects

In many studies, people or animals might become sick or injured incidental to participation, or by factors irrelevant to participation. In most cases, negative outcomes for participating subjects is rare. Nevertheless, you must maximally safeguard subjects from physical, mental, and emotional pain and suffering as a consequence of participation. Applicants should comment on the potential for stress, the potential for psychological harm due to inadvertent disclosure of the very fact of participating, and certainly harm from disclosure of their individual data, which you promise to keep confidential.

Because some clinical trials that are testing new treatments include subjects with terminal prognoses, clinical trials have special criteria to ensure patient safety. Human subject researchers must be aware that there are reporting requirements for adverse events (Sect. 5.4.2), and the procedures you will follow should be spelled out in step-by-step manner using the new 2018 consolidated *PHS Human Subjects and Clinical Trials Form E*. The new form consolidates information that used to appear in a variety of application sections, was often redundant (especially when clinical trials were involved), and increased the likelihood of inadequate communication of safeguards, in part because protections took up space in the page-limited research plan. The new form allows greater detail in describing human protections. Detailed instructions are described in the latest Research Instructions For NIH.[1]

There are studies that are exempt from human-subjects protection requirements Yours is probably NOT one of them. Most research routinely conducted in educational settings that examine/evaluate normal educational practices are exempt. Survey and/or educational test research involving participants over age 18 under conditions of anonymity are exempt. Some political research examining public office incumbents or candidates are exempt. Secondary analysis of publicly-available data, documents, records, and specimens for which subject identities have been removed are exempt. However, most secondary analyses are not exempt because even when identities are coded and not known to the investigator, personal characteristics obtained for moderator/mediator analysis might identify the only over-50 female in a specific department. Research evaluating the public benefit of service programs are exempt as is research examining the appeal of certain foods to consumers is exempt. It is our strong suggestion that you contact your organization's Institutional Review Board (IRB) to clearly understand requirements since non-exempt protocols should be submitted to your human subjects review committee before applying for a grant or contract. An IRB is required to approve and monitor all human subjects research conducted by an institution.[2]

Undue risk to human subjects or experimental animal subjects is normally a show-stopper for a grant application Ensure that you address every item on your application form. If you think the rules do not apply, it is prudent to explain why you think they do not apply. It also makes sense to get input from a program official at the funding institution. If your judgment is wrong, you might not even get as far as peer review.

The use of animals in research is in steep decline, but animals still have a significant role in research such as determining medication effectiveness. Genetic and genomic research is increasingly using animals to refine gene editing procedures. Table 4.2 lists the NIH criteria for using animals in research. They normally apply

---

[1] https://grants.nih.gov/grants/how-to-apply-application-guide/forms-e/research-forms-e.pdf

[2] https://www.hhs.gov/ohrp/register-irbs-and-obtain-fwas/irb-registration/index.html has more IRB information.

Table 4.2   NIH criteria for using animals in research[a]

Rationale for animal use and consideration of alternatives
Justification for the choice of species and number of animals
Research procedures involving animals
Procedures to minimize pain and distress
Animal living conditions and veterinary care
Names and qualifications of personnel who will perform work with animals
Method of euthanasia; and endpoint criteria

[a]Source: NIH Office of animal welfare [https://grants.nih.gov/grants/policy/air/policy.htm]

to any funding institution or agency. NIH offers extensive guidance on human and animal protection.[3]

It is often a good idea, when appropriate, to discuss any government licenses, regular inspections and certifications, and put them in your appendices. If you have used animals in previous projects, explain any adverse events experienced and how your lab and vivarium are equipped to respond. Lastly, we live in an era in which some militant animal rights groups invade vivaria and recklessly release animals to disrupt research and/or to "save" the animals. Often, such invasions wind up killing animals and/or requiring euthanasia. It also can wipe out hundreds of thousands of research dollars and delay life-saving information and interventions. Thus, it is a good idea to comment on vivarium security, especially after hours.

4.2.5   Commitment for Laboratory & Equipment

We noted earlier, the odds of getting funded improve when your institution offers significant support. Things like facility awards or other recognition, gratis laboratory and/or office space, computing equipment, as well as laboratory equipment provided by your institution lowers risk and lowers cost.

It might be that you will need to rely on outside support such as specimen assay services or MRI scanners. It is not sufficient to say; "The University Medical Center will provide access to the required MRI." Reviewers know that expensive equip-

---

[3] Sites to visit for human subjects: https://humansubjects.nih.gov/; https://www.nsf.gov/pubs/policydocs/pappguide/nsf16001/gpg_2.jsp#IID8. For animal subjects go to https://grants.nih.gov/grants/olaw/olaw.htm; https://www.nsf.gov/pubs/policydocs/pappguide/nsf16001/gpg_2.jsp#IID7

ment in hospitals is in high demand, and often is booked weeks in advance. To dispel all doubt, obtain a letter of commitment from the hospital that X number of hours of MRI access will be made available at Y cost – better yet, at no cost. The same applies, for example, to colliders, large lasers, etc. **Without details, a letter of support committing resources carries little weight**.

In our opinion, you cannot include too many letters of support (LOSs). LOSs from hospitals, clinics, and other organizations where you intend to recruit research subjects count a lot, your dean's support, statements of enthusiasm from leaders in the field are helpful. LOSs should also be obtained from any organization within or outside your institution that will be supplying essential equipment access and/or lab access, space, analysis, or any other critical service or support should be included.

Quality LOSs are easiest to obtain if you draft major parts of the letter so it can be changed for signature. Appendix D provides an outline for LOS content that might be helpful.

4.2.6   Commitment from the Subject Pool Source

It is easy to overlook where and how human subjects will be recruited. Usually an investigator knows about a target-rich setting in which to recruit. If human subjects are involved, the following questions should be addressed: How can you assure reviewers that you have access to your recruitment setting(s)? What procedures will you use to ensure adequate protection of the human subjects that will be approached to participate? **What assurances will be made to potential subjects** (in writing) regarding their safety, any potential risks to participation, and of course, protection of their data and identity?

If your target subjects are medical patients, recruiting can be a sensitive process as you risk violating their privacy even if they do not participate. For example, imagine that you have Hepatitis C and some stranger approaches you to join a Hep C study. The patient might think; "How did they know I have Hep C? My doctor must have breached my confidentiality." Thus, trust in your assertions of confidentiality already have been undermined by your recruitment attempt. **Describing how recruiting referrals will be made** (usually with a direct hand-off from the patient's attending physician), will dispel concerns about this issue. Ideally, the referral agent should alert patients of pending contact and ascertain their willingness to be contacted before introducing them to the recruiter.

4.2.7   Cost Versus Benefit: The Level of Effort Concept

A significant part of research planning is assembling a budget. So how can you be sure your budget is, and will, appear to be appropriate? One approach that can be helpful is used frequently by the Department of Defense: the notion of "level of effort" (LOE). **LOE is the total cost of effort and resources to obtain**

information within a specified period of time. The more time and resources needed; the higher will be the project LOE. Most reviewers and funders weigh a project's LOE against *validity* (required or promised), *problem importance*, and the *urgency* for the resulting deliverables (reports, algorithms, prototypes, etc.). Because LOE is a concept, it is in the mind of the reviewer; not a mathematical formula. Thus, it is subject to bias and misinformation. What you put in your application can reduce bias and clarify information.

Normally, it should take an <u>average LOE</u> to get a <u>meaningfully useful</u> result given the time and resources requested. It should take an <u>above-average LOE</u> (higher cost) to get a <u>definitive</u> result given the time and resources requested; and, it should take a <u>huge LOE</u> to get a definitive result <u>urgently</u> such as developing medications to treat and protect against emergent epidemics. Even under circumstances of high urgency, cost remains a factor.

We have observed that most review panels evaluate project budgets in terms of LOE even if they do not use that term. The question in the mind of both funding institutions and reviewers is: **"Does the LOE match the value, importance, precision, and urgency of the proposed study?** If LOE is lower than the proposed cost, the study will appear to be *over-budgeted*. If the LOE is higher than its cost, the study will likely appear to be *under-budgeted*, and risk running out of support before the project is completed. When considering grant applications, LOE also has bearing on the capacity of the investigator, research group, and facilities to accomplish the study on time.

4.2.8 Ways to Lower Costs: Recruit Investors & Take Your Time

One of the best ways to lower project costs is to share the risk. Banks often reduce risk by selling some of their loans to other banks in exchange for reduced loss and lower profits. The same situations apply to federal grants. Government agencies (local, state, or federal) and foundations with mission overlap look to each other at times to share project risks. Of course, in the event of success, co-funders share the credit for supporting your institution's research. Your institution might be willing to contribute support by providing resources like staff support, cost-sharing, or reducing its overhead to reduce the cost of your study and thereby reduce the risk for the funding institution(s). When Tom and Carl were at NIH, if there was a great project that came out of review with a very low score but a very high price tag, they would usually try to reduce their institute's cost by "by shopping the project around" to other NIH institutes for co-funding. If the costs were still too high, they would call colleagues in other agencies and private foundations. Once, Tom even took a project to the White House for help.[4] Lastly, if co-funding cannot cover project costs, a PO

---

[4] In case you're wondering, the WH, Tom's last resort, turned him down; but the fact that he went that far, convinced his institute director to fund the entire project – happy ending.

will usually contact the Principal Investigator and try to negotiate modifications such as extending the project timeline across more fiscal years, cutting out nonessential subprojects (arms) that could be studied in a smaller project later, or asking for the PI's institution to contribute more resources.

If public safety, national security, or the economy is not at high risk, then a smaller budget request spread out over several years makes sense because it reduces the annual cost to the funding institution. Lower costs enable funding a greater number of projects, while at the same time supporting less-urgent, albeit worthwhile, projects like fellowships. Likewise, exploratory studies have a high risk of discovering that there is nothing of great importance, even though learning that might inform future research. For example, suppose you can only expect to get a <u>meaningfully and useful result</u> for $100 K in 2 years using an NIH small grant (R03). Alternatively, you might be confident that you can make a case that a <u>more definitive result</u> could be obtained in 3 years at a cost of $200 K with an extra year to collect more data. Applying for a small 3-year R01 at $65 K/year might make your application seem more competitive than use of the smaller, shorter-term mechanism because the deliverables (your reported results) will have greater perceived value. Both approaches have relatively low costs, but the funding agency might be more interested in getting a bigger bang for the buck so to speak by funding the longer study.

4.3   Application Forms

Application Forms

- Register w/Funders
- Complete All Assurances
- Complete Application Forms
- Institutional (SO) Approval
- Grants.gov Submission

Once you have a solid outline describing your project, it's time to start the bureaucratic process of completing application forms. As we said earlier, your institution should have experts to guide you with completing your application materials. They may have software to help compute budgets that can pop the numbers into the budget pages. If for some reason this is not the case, many universities post guidance on the Internet for faculty to use. You might look initially for guidance there. In addition, government websites and most nongovernment agencies offer explicit step-by-step application guidance.

4.3.1   Application Forms: Writing & the Train of Thought

We always advise grant applicants to focus on telling a good story well Your primary goal is to engage your reviewers' interest in your project. You want to create a mindset that leads reviewers to think things like: "Wow! This is something that needs to be done." As well as LOE - "These seem to be the right hypotheses and the right controls for the right price." You cannot accomplish this positive reaction if you periodically interrupt your reviewer's *Train of Thought* or put the train's caboose in front of the engine.

Ideally, you want that *Train of Thought* to leave your "Aims" station and steam along the tracks in the direction you laid them, moving at a constant pace, until comfortably arriving at a favorable review and a positive funding decision. You also want to avoid distractions along the way such as, unscheduled stops, slowdowns to make noisy tight turns, and most definitely having to wander from car to car looking for things.

Aims As mentioned earlier, your research project aims set the stage. They tell passengers on your *Train of Thought* where they are going, and alert them to noteworthy points of interest along the way. The most common problem we have seen is putting the caboose before the engine. This occurs when you start with a meandering literature review before announcing the destination – your aims.

Sidetracks When your reviewers board your *Train of Thought,* you don't want to sidetrack them. If you go off on a tangent (e.g., discuss non-essential literature), it is the same as pulling the train onto a siding to allow anther train to pass by. Readers might have to re-read sections of your application to get back on track. The best way to avoid sidetracks is to include enough information that reviewers will accept your point or rationale as reasonable/valid, then move on.

Sudden Lurches Lurches occur when you write a sentence that doesn't makes sense. Lurches cause the passengers on your *Train of Thought* to experience unexpected confusion, requiring them to try to stop, re-read, and try to make sense of what you just said. Having others review your application before submission can help to identify missing words, choppy paragraphs, run-on sentences, and under/over punctuation.

Slowdowns Slowdowns occur when your *Train of Thought* must make a logical transition or spell out details such as computational formulae. Keep in mind the adage that sometimes "a picture is worth a thousand words." A graphic figure or table might help to maintain the reading pace. You can always put formulae in the appendix if it is not essential to building your case. *However, if a figure takes up more space than 1000 words, weigh the pros and cons of using a figure or table.*

Stuff Left at the Station When embarking on any trip, you must make decisions about what to take with you. Leave something essential behind, and you will have to make do without. Errors of omission tend to be more common because space is limited in many application forms. Thus, you have to pack your ideas into a tight bundle of thoughts. However, over-editing risks tossing the proverbial baby out with the bathwater. Sentences can seem choppy and/or hard to follow, and you might have inadvertently omitted a key word. As reviewers follow along on your *Train of Thought*, each time there is information that they need to know but cannot find in your application (errors of omission), your score will go up a little.

Keep in mind, that sometimes you have no choice but to leave something behind. Always be aware of when you choose do that and weigh strategically which things to omit that are least likely to drive up your score.

Derailments You risk derailing a reviewer's *Train of Thought* whenever you require them to hunt for explanations of terms or acronyms that were inadequate or last mentioned too many pages earlier. If you introduce an acronym on page 1, but do not use it again until the bottom of page 4, and you have used 4 or 5 acronyms already, spell it out again. Don't make the readers have to PgUp◯ or flip back looking for it. At that point – you have derailed their *Train of Thought*. Worse, if you failed to introduce the acronym or explain a term, you have also annoyed them – and your score goes up more. Here are some proven suggestions for keeping your application on track:

- Exclude non-essential hypotheses and aims.
- Avoid including marginal literature – *stay focused on literature that justifies your aims.*
- Avoid more budget detail than requested – *risks surgical budget cuts.*
- Use acronyms and coined terms sparingly – *not all reviewers may be in your field.*
- Re-introduce acronyms or terminology if not used for several pages.
- Don't include biosketches of marginal team members – *raises concerns about who's doing the research.*
- Use equations sparingly unless certain that all reviewers will understand them.
- A proven way to identify sidetracks and derailments is by sitting in the room while people read your draft application. *If you see them flip back – immediately ask why.*
- Get as many people as possible to review and critique your draft application.

4.3.2 Register with the Funding Institution as Soon as You Decide to Apply

Not all federal agencies or other funding institutions require advanced notice or special registration to apply for a grant. However, many government agencies have registration requirements beyond that for Grants.Gov because there are often laws and regulations specific to that agency which have unique requirements. For example, in DOD, security clearances and nondisclosure agreements (NDAs) are often essential to do contract research. In many cases, NIH especially, there is mandatory training on select regulations that is required of all applicants. Most, if not all, of this training can be done online, but must be completed before submitting. Guidance on registration requirements can be found in FOAs, but it is wise to check the funding institution's website.

4.3.3   Complete and Submit All Assurances Ahead of Formal Submission

Assurances are certifications by an applicant, normally included with the application, indicating that you and your institution are in compliance with, or that it will abide by, various requirements when awarded a Federal grant. Assurances can be specific to an FOA such as a request for applications or generally for all awardees. Human subjects and animal protection policy adherence are examples of typical assurances. Your organization should be helpful in their completion.

4.3.4   Complete All Application Forms

Applicants for federal grants go to Grants.Gov to submit applications online. In 2002, Grants.Gov was initiated by the Office of Management and Budget as part of a partisan-inspired effort to make government function more like a business. The goal in creating Grants.Gov and the SF424 application form was to create one site and one form to apply for any federal grant. Although Grants.Gov sounded like a great idea, it overlooked the diversity of missions and complexity of vetting applications unique to many agencies. Diverse missions and technology often require specialized information beyond the SF424. For NIH applications, HHS created ASSIST as an alternative to Grants.Gov with the intention of being less confusing. Your FOA might require using ASSIST.

The SF424 form and embedded PHS 398 can seem a bit crazy, because it is designed to support the vetting process; not to make it easy for you to explain what you want to do. As a rule, never take any section of a form page lightly. Complete each section. If it does not apply, complete the section and explain why it does not apply.

4.3.5   Preparing to Submit Your Application

Once your application is complete – all "i's" are dotted and "t's" crossed, it is ready for peer review. You may at that point submit the application to your university AOR, or if the AOR has delegated that responsibility to you, you may upload it yourself. But before you do that, are you really ready? If time permits, you might want to send the final package around to a few colleagues – just in case you missed something. Given the size of your application, do not be surprised if your feedback is terse, superficial, or even late. It takes time to review a complete grant application package, and your colleagues have other priorities. Some PIs farm out just key sections.

Some research institutions quietly pay experienced outside experts a consulting fee to provide a quick and thorough pre-review critique of their draft applications before they submit it to NIH or other funding institutions. Some limit their review request to just the research plan. Others include the entire application package. In case you were wondering, yes, it appears to be a very successful strategy. Given the cost and lost time to revise and resubmit, paid reviews might catch omissions or errors easily fixed before submission that would drive up your score in review. Usually paid reviewers are chosen because they have experience as review panel members and/or are retired POs. Of course, you need to be careful about whom you pay to pre-review an application since that reviewer will have to recuse themselves from reviewing and scoring your application for the government. Keep in mind that retirees and emeritus faculty often lack rigid schedules and might enjoy engaging in professional activities now and then if invited to do so.

4.3.6   Rushing to Catch the Gravy Train

Unsolicited RPGs   What if the clock is ticking and you are not sure that you can make the RFA/RFP submission deadline in time? Rushing your application to meet an FOA submission deadline risks submitting an insufficiently developed application package, and not being scored. Initially waiting for 3 or 4 additional months until the next review cycle might save 6 months spent waiting to receive and review the summary statement to revise and resubmit. If you miss an RFA deadline, it is usually straightforward to revise and submit an unsolicited RPG to a program FOA.

4.3.7   Obtain Your Institution's Approval to Submit Your Application and Submit

Once you are satisfied that you are as ready as you can be – submit the application prior to the published deadline internally to meet any final university requirements including approvals. Then either the AOR or a person designated by him to the funding agency (maybe you) pushes the "Enter" button. But, as we mentioned earlier, that might result in an immediate rejection for format errors, or even days later for some other error. Stay available for the next week just in case.

Even if the Grants.Gov software does not detect an error, you are not out of the woods. Many agencies, NIH for example, have humans look at all applications to ensure that they are responsive to the FOA, contain no obvious omissions such as human protection and conflicts of interest statements. They also check that the applicant institution, the PI, and other key personnel are qualified, have completed any required pre-registrations, and all required training and other certifications are on file. Only after technical clearance will your application be accepted by an agency's funding institution (e.g., an NIH IC). It might take a week to catch a problem, so a last-minute submission leaves insufficient time to fix any application technical issues.

Here are a few of the more common rejection triggers:

- The DUNS number does not match your institution's DUNS number (typo?). [Note: All grants carry the applicant institution's unique Dun & Bradstreet D-U-N-S Number]
- You inadvertently uploaded a virus in a file attachment.
- Attachments do not follow the proper naming convention, and/or package elements (files) exceeded the word count or page length.
- PROJECT TITLES may not exceed 200 characters including spaces or you included a forbidden character like a question mark "?". [Note: More on title length in Sect. 5.1]
- The application was submitted after the deadline for receiving applications.
- You registered with Grants.Gov but not the funding agency.
- Your Grants.Gov username is not authorized by your institution's AOR to submit applications from your organization.

Chapter 5
Application Content

Application Content

- Project & Information
- Cover Letter
- Research Plan
- Sample
- Collaboration/Team
- Appendices

This chapter builds on the previous discussion of the application process and focuses attention on the actual content of your application – what to include and what to omit. By discussing the National Institutes of Health application, we will cover nearly all of the application content issues facing most grant applications. Some funding institutions, foundations especially, can have very unstructured applications. Following the NIH path will often strengthen what you present, thus improving your odds of a favorable decision.

New investigators often ask POs what a completed grant application looks like. There are some examples downloadable from https://www.niaid.nih.gov/grants-contracts/sample-applications. In addition, many university websites post successful faculty applications which can be downloaded and examined. We recommend you ask mentors and senior colleagues for a peek at their past successful applications. Looking at an entire application package can help you to see how everything hangs together. However, it would be wise not to use them as a rigid template. It might cramp your writing style or lead to a confusing organization. Lastly, because the government changes the rules periodically, you should always check in with your grants office and ask for help identifying any recent funding notices that might communicate changes in policy or procedures. Sometimes applicants call in with questions, and NIH publishes notes of clarification.

Keep in mind that as we pointed out in Chap. 1, all researchers are trained to do everything necessary to prepare a grant application, as part of their doctoral training. When you proposed your masters thesis and doctoral dissertation, you probably prepared concept papers to get a sense of your committee's support for your idea. You then drafted detailed proposals (just like a grant or contract application), and it was reviewed by a panel of experts – your faculty. You received feedback and made changes in your approach to meet faculty committee concerns – just as you would

© The Author(s), under exclusive license to Springer Nature Switzerland AG 2019   55
T. F. Hilton, C. G. Leukefeld, *Grantsmanship for New Investigators*,
SpringerBriefs in Public Health, https://doi.org/10.1007/978-3-030-01301-1_5

if your grant application did not score low enough. Those concerns might have been statistical or design-related, how you addressed human subjects protection, and all of the things that grant applicants encounter when starting their career to become an independent investigator. Once approved, you then implemented your research plans under the watchful eye of your major professor(s) (much as you would rely upon a grant consultant or Co-I) and drafted a publishable manuscript. The entire graduate school process familiarized you with how government regulations and scientific standards work to ensure sound science and humane treatment of humans and animals in research. Alas, they did not require that you use a counter-intuitive format. The government has accountants, lawyers, and scientists reviewing your application, and this results in forms being compartmented to facilitate review.

5.1 Project and Applicant Information

As previously mentioned, the SF424 is boilerplate more useful to entitlement applications than for grants. Thus, NIH tacks on the SF424, its own lengthy PHS application Form 398. That is where you start to build your case to the review panel. The application process might not seem like science. It isn't. It's salesmanship. It is where you and your institution present evidence of your human and technical resources. The first page must stand alone as the summary of your application to NIH. As such, it is essential that your title and abstract nicely summarize your project. It may be the only document some funding decision-makers or Congressional staff might look at. There is an annotated version of the NIH SF424 (and PHS398) online form at https://grants.nih.gov/grants/ElectronicReceipt/files/Annotated_Forms_General_FORMS-E.pdf which might help you navigate the process.

Titles are very important NIH accepts titles of up to 200 characters. However, strategically, your title should clearly relate what you are studying, and possibly why in fewer than 81 characters including spaces because some databases only show the first 80 characters of the title. Your title should be written at a level your grandmother can understand. Crafting a good title is time well-spent because your shorter title becomes your project's "handle" when people discuss it during review, vetting, and after your award.

An overly long title risks looking like this: "**A SNIP analysis of the venom of the Brazilian tree frog Osteocephalus Subtilis: A**" The system will omit the rest of the title beyond 80 characters which included: "*possible vaccine for pancreatic cancer.*" A congressional staffer might wonder why studying an "*Osteocephalus Subtilis: A*" is worth a \$2 M price tag. Your local newspaper might headline: *University researcher gets \$two million grant to study tree frogs in Brazil.* Not good. Your NIH handle will likely become "The Tree Frog Study" and NOT the "Cancer Vaccine Study." And even your PO will despise you for all the time they had to spend answering post-award public inquiries. Similarly, being too clever can also get you unwanted attention. Using the same fictional study: "**A SNIP in vines**

saves lives in time: How Brazilian tree frogs might cure cancer." This title begs questions rather than provides information. Snipping down vines to harvest tree frogs can cure cancer?

A better title might be: "**The effect of tree frog venom on pancreatic cancer cells: A SNIP analysis.**" Use the same title for SF424 as you use for your embedded form PHS398. Otherwise you risk and error upon submission.

After your title, your abstract is the next segment of your application that will be read the most. Your abstract and your score may be all that is read by those who can influence your funding. Thus, you want to pack as much information in it as possible to ensure that: (a) it will appear to be a good investment by anybody who reads it, including Capitol Hill, and (b) it highlights the main value to both the agency (Institute or Center) mission and science generally.

In summary:

- The title is the main reference for discussing your application at all meetings
- The title can get you unwanted attention if you get too windy or too clever
- The abstract should enable congressional staff and others to understand your grant

5.1.1   Detailed Budget (First Year) and Projected Budget

Your budget says to reviewers and funding institutions far more than you might think. Along with your key personnel section, your budget is a reviewer's best indication of your planned *level of effort* (Sect. 4.2.7). It relates who is doing what for the project, when, where, and for how long. Figure 5.1 shows a redacted budget form for an NIH R01. By defining roles, the budget pages set the stage for reviewing your biosketches. Look it over. If anything leaps out at you as unusual, like $40 K for copying services, make sure that you did not mean to type $4 K. But, if it is $40 K, explain why the amount is unusually high. If you do not, expect a recommendation for reduced award. Once that happens, it is far trickier to restore the funds.

It is best to describe the necessary equipment, supplies, facilities down to the specs, and include any fees for use. For example, there may be technician services from people not on your team, and those should be factored into your costs on your budget pages.

There are two kinds of budget formats used by NIH: detailed and modular. These are described in detail at https://grants.nih.gov/grants/how-to-apply-application-guide/format-and-write/develop-your-budget.htm#modular. Basically, for grants under $250 K/year you submit a modular budget which contains less detail than a larger research grant. Regardless of the form, you will likely have to draft a detailed budget in order to determine how many $25 K modules to request in a modular format (1–10). Even when detailed budgets are required, you normally limit details to year #1.

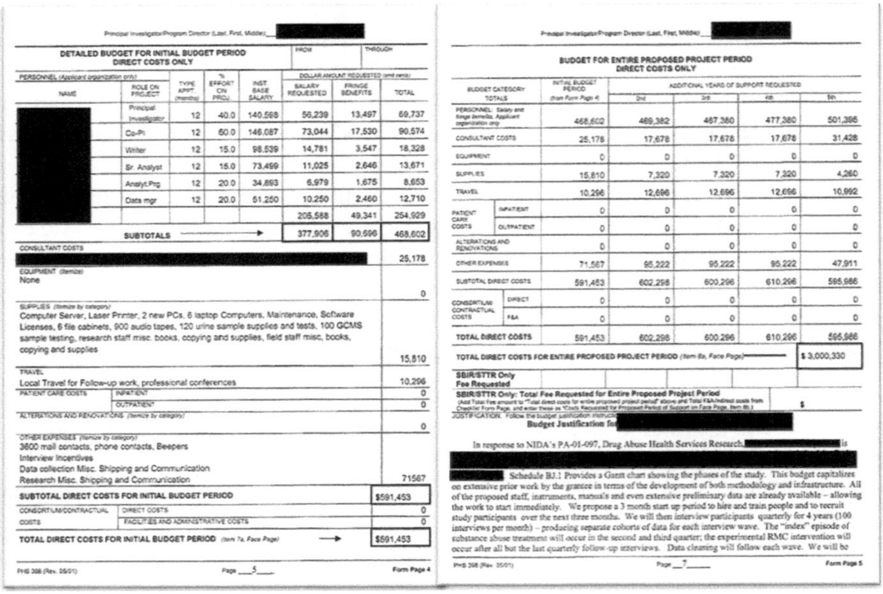

Fig. 5.1 A redacted budget form for an R01

A big reason for a detailed budget is to help the funding institution accounting personnel. Most of the complexities of starting a project get worked out during the initial budget year. For example, support contracts and rental arrangements are established, equipment needs are accessed, technical support staff are recruited, and certifications are filed.

Sometimes, detailed budgets are required for more than the initial year. The FOA will describe any additional detailed budgets and their periodicity. In extra-large projects, the request for applications might specify budget details required of applicants that differ from the norm. Working up the budget will confront you with questions you might not have considered, so it is prudent to draft your research plan (Sect. 5.4.3) before tackling your budget.

The Budget Justification page is a narrative and can run as many pages as needed. This is an often- overlooked salesmanship opportunity to reiterate your research strategy. There are usually sections which include: (a) senior/key personnel, (b) other personnel, (c) equipment, (d) travel, and (e) other costs. You start by detailing the roles and responsibilities of each of the key personnel. Key Personnel are listed by name and role. Use one paragraph to describe each. Anybody you name must have an included biosketch (next section) and their letter of support (Sect. 5.5.3) reflecting their commitment to the success of the project. Other Personnel are usually technical support staff who should be named. They may be listed as TBA (To Be Assigned). This often includes separate costs for students as graduate research assistants and postdocs when allowed. Reviewers check for these sorts of things.

Equipment should include computers, lab equipment, software, and measurement tools. Explain what the equipment will be used for. Don't leave reviewers guessing. Travel includes travel for data collection, coordination meetings, as well as conferences and other presentations where you will disseminate interim and final results. Include how you arrived at the costs, and who you anticipate traveling. Other Costs include supplies, rentals, services, software licenses, servers, and incentive payments to human subjects. Again, explain your rationale for paying subjects – citing precedents can sometimes be helpful if incentives are pricey.

In summary, your budget:

- Indicates who is doing what and their level of effort in time and cost
- Includes justifications for team roles and resources requested
- Describes roles and implies needed expertise
- Justifies resources requested including travel and travel to do what
- Justifies any large amounts – $10 K for phone calls? $75 K for travel?

5.1.2 Key Personnel

An ideal strategy for completing this section of your application is to make it read like a university recruiting brochure designed to convince parents to invest their children's future and their tuition money by taking advantage of the world-class faculty and their cutting-edge laboratories. Analogously, you are trying to convince a group of senior colleagues and a funding institution to invest grant money in you as well as your institutions' research program.

We also suggest omitting as key personnel those who do not specifically add to the project. For NIH applications, you are asked to specifically describe the role and responsibilities of each staff member along with a brief biography explaining their expertise and how each person contributes to the project. Minor roles such as technicians can be listed as To Be Assigned (TBA).

5.1.3 Biographical Sketches (PI and Key Personnel)

Biographical sketches (biosketches) justify your budget request, include justifications for team member roles, and establish expertise related to the project; not expertise in general. If you are beginning your research career, you might not have many publications, much less germane to the project. In general, reviewers base their expectations on the seniority of the person filling out the biosketch. An applicant or key person with one publication may summarize the key finding of the paper and its importance in a short contribution. An applicant or key person with no publications might describe their efforts on prior projects and papers that they worked on e.g.," I used this method; I conducted the literature review for this paper, etc."

A good biosketch section introduces the cast of characters to your reviewer audience. We have found that a good strategy is to introduce them like a movie trailer: "Starring: Joyce PI and Barry Consultant, Co-staring: James Psychometrician, Mary MRI Expert, with Bill Numbercruncher; and introducing newcomer Field Interviewer." Each biosketch has a maximum of five pages to present the expertise of each key person – two or three is common. The goal of each is to explain, first-person, what their role will be, and what experience and qualifications make them particularly well-suited for the project. Include relevant experience, education, training, and publications. It is best not to cite papers irrelevant to the person's role on the project. Those you can summarize.

Your biosketch strategy should be to establish your expertise as well as coinvestigators and your lab/field staff. These sketches present an essential justification for your budget. You want reviewers to view you and your team as being well-qualified including training and experience to achieve everything in your research plan. Again, you want to emphasize capabilities relevant to the project.

Biosketches are available as an online fillable form that includes four sections:

A. Personal Statement. Describe first-person why you are well-suited with your training, technical expertise, previous research, and with whom you might have worked. You are allowed to cite up to four refereed publications or other research experience.
B. Positions and Honors. In chronological order, list professional awards/honors. New investigators and students can include: postdoctorates, professional licenses, medical board certifications, scholarships, and fellowships.
C. Contributions to Science. Describe up to five of your most significant contributions. You may cite up to four publications for each. Start with a brief historical background/context that frames the scientific problem; describe the findings, characterize their influence on the field, what your role was and anything else that builds your case for relevant expertise.
D. Additional Information. Prior and current research support and/or scholastic performance in the case of students.

Most funding institutions requiring biosketches offer appropriate examples such as this one from NIH: http://grants.nih.gov/grants/forms/biosketch-sample.docx

Strategic Caveat Only include material relevant to the project aims. Reviewers do not care that your number cruncher did a post-doc at Stanford in a topic not relevant to your study. Thus, make sure team members order their citations from most to least relevant to your project. Tom reviewed an application from a PhD who had changed fields from mechanical engineering to biology. The biosketch cited over 100 engineering publications but offered no information regarding his qualifications to conduct the biological study for which he was applying. It was not scored.

Curriculum Vitae In addition to the descriptions of specific contributions and documentation, **applicants can include an Internet link** to a full list of their published work on a publicly available digital database such as provided by the National Library of Medicine's National Center for Biotechnology Information[1] **MyBibliography** or The Science Experts Network Curriculum Vitae (SciENcv). As **SciENcv** is the federal standard, it would be prudent to use it rather than competing sites. If you include this link do not expect reviewers to bother checking your full CV, because they are not required to. Thus, put your best foot forward when listing publications. They should be the best you have that are related to the project.

5.1.4 Resources

In describing your performances site(s), build the best case that you can. Include things like history of accomplishment, years of experience, diversity of perspective, unique facilities and equipment, anything that will help to establish that you will be doing research in an ideal setting. It also reassures reviewers that you have ample backup on tap (experts and equipment) in the event that unforeseen barriers are encountered.

The Resources Page is unstructured. You do not need to talk about staplers and paper, but you do want to identify the relevant facilities to be used. Many applications devote a paragraph each to: laboratory, clinical, animal, computer, office, and other. If appropriate, indicate their capacities, pertinent capabilities, relative proximity and extent of availability to the project. Describe only those resources that are directly applicable to the proposed work. Provide information describing the Other Resources available to the project (e.g., machine shop, electronic shop) and the extent to which they would be available to the project if needed. If you are not likely to need a machine shop, even if you have access to one, it risks being distracting reviewers to mention it.

Another salesmanship opportunity relates to describing how the scientific environment in which the research will be conducted adds to the probability of success (e.g., institutional support, physical resources, and intellectual rapport). Describe any unique features of the environment, especially things, as appropriate, like cyclotrons, MRI, CAT, and other costly equipment as well as the experience/reputation of the technical team that will operate it. Describe any special facilities for working with biohazards or other potentially dangerous substances. If there are multiple performance sites, describe the resources available at each site.

For Early Stage Investigators, support and availability of organized peer groups; administrative management, and protected time from teaching and faculty responsibilities also should be mentioned.

---

[1] https://www.ncbi.nlm.nih.gov/account/?back_url=https%3A%2F%2Fwww.ncbi.nlm.nih.gov%2Fsites%2Fmyncbi%2F

5.2   Cover Letter

In the event that your application gets misassigned or otherwise goes adrift in the NIH or larger federal agency review system (which can occur for several days or even weeks before being discovered) your optional *cover letter* offers navigation tips to the receiving agency department and the SRO assigned to coordinate peer review of your application. Federal systems can get overburdened, or somebody (you even) might click the wrong key – then whammo! Your application goes to the wrong agency, institute, center, or office.

Cover letters are for SROs only. Peer reviewers do not see them. The content of your letter should state the FOA title and number. If multiple agencies/institutes sponsor the FOA, indicate to which you are applying. It is also prudent to mention the name of any PO with whom you have been interacting about the application to help get it assigned to a sympathetic branch.

You should also use the PHS Application Request Form to request a suitable Initial Review Group (IRG) panel (also called a Study Section). Peer review panel members cannot access this page. If there is someone who in your opinion has a conflict of interest or strong personal bias against you and is a standing member on the review panel to which you anticipate your application being assigned, you may mention the basis for your concern in your PHS Application Request Form. The SRO will take it under advisement but may not necessarily exclude that individual since researchers can disagree. Tom has seen SRO's delete a score if the review appeared to be biased. Keep in mind that your score is the average of the entire panel. Outlier reviewers must submit a written justification for their extreme score, as it is NIH practice that panelists vote between the lowest and highest scores of the primary reviewers.

5.3   Research Plan

The research plan is the meat and potatoes of your application. Ideally, it is your chance to describe your great idea for the proposed study in its entirety. This where you want to be engineer of your ***Train of Thought.*** It explains what you aim to do, the rationale for doing it, describes how aims and hypotheses derive logically from previous research or preliminary data, identifies the key hypotheses that will help improve understanding of the topic, lines up the sample, describes what you intend to measure with which tools, and how you plan to analyze your data. It sets the entire project in the context of an outstanding institution with impressive scientists, technical support, and a history of success.

The research plan is your strategic, "brief-but-spectacular,"[2] approach to your study. It should describe tactics to overcome scientific and logistic barriers, plans to

---

[2] To parody the regular PBS News Hour "My Brief But Spectacular" segment.

minimize unanticipated problems and surprises, as well as present a team of highly trained researchers and specialists to help you carry out and achieve aims that will advance science as well as the funding institutions mission. Avoid hype, but be enthusiastic.

Keep in mind that your application has two audiences: the majority of reviewers who will probably not be familiar with your techniques or specific area of interest, and a smaller number (likely your primary/principal reviewers) who will be familiar. They are all accomplished researchers.

The remainder of this chapter overviews the application elements from a strategic perspective. As we have already pointed out, your institution has staff with experience in ensuring the proper format and administrative information are addressed.

5.3.1   Introduction Page (Resubmissions or Revisions Only)

If resubmitting or seeking a competitive renewal of a completed grant, you are required to include an introduction section. For resubmissions, this section should explain how each concern or criticism of the review panel is addressed in the resubmission. As some of the same reviewers are likely to look at your resubmission, it is prudent not to argue that an earlier review criticism was inappropriate – overlooked a pivotal study, missed a nuance of the analysis plan, or some other "reasonable" situation that you have clarified in your revised application. Swallow your pride and address each concern – just fix it. If an application is for the renewal of a grant, this section should overview the accomplishments of the previous project.

5.3.2   Research Aims and Strategy (Typical R01/RPG Outline)

Your *Aims Page* provides a roadmap for where you want to go with your project. **The *Aims Page* of your application creates a framework and mindset for reviewers.** As Sect. 4.3.4 described, it lays the tracks that will guide the *Train of Thought* for reviewers. Think of your introductory paragraph as the cognitive glue to which reviewers might stick the information you provide in the next 4–6 paragraphs as you describe your project. If reviewers are at paragraph 5 and are still unsure about the purpose of your project, their *Train of Thought* is still in the station! The rest of the application better be spectacular. The subsequent sections/topics are common sense, but nevertheless, skipping or inadequately communicating your intent for each is the main reason grants go unscored in review. Note: Do not duplicate information collected in the new 2018 PHS Human Subjects and Clinical Trials form (E).

In nearly all cases, applicants whose *Aims Page* beats around the bush, putting #2 (the why) before #1 (the what), risks annoying their reviewers right off the bat. In the first sentence, stipulate what the project is supposed to do and how you intended

Table 5.1 Essential elements of your Aims page

1. *This project requests $####K for # years to... (aims in 1 sentence). The **problem is**... what is **not known** is ...*
2. *Our **long-term goal** is ... our **central hypothesis** is that... our **rationale** is based on... this project is **relevant** because... (how it advances science/practice)*
Our central hypotheses will be tested by pursuing the following aims:...
3. ***Aim #1** is to...*
4. ***Aim #2** is to...*
5. ***Aim #3** is to...*
6. *This project is **innovative** because... our **research environment** will ensure the success of this project because... the **expected outcomes** include... we think this research is **significant** because... Results should have a **positive impact** on... (impact aligned with institute/agency mission)*

to do it. In the same paragraph, you can mention the level of effort (time and resources) associated with the project so readers get a sense of the scope, magnitude, and duration of your proposed project. Alas, the majority of applicants dribble this level of effort information across multiple paragraphs, and thereby miss an opportunity to help guide the reviewers' *Train of Thought*. Remember, those reviewing and vetting your application will all be asking the same question: "Is this project worth it?" **Rest assured, the expert review panel already knows the literature you are about to present as justification of your request**, so don't bore them with numerous paragraphs of familiar "why" information before getting around to telling them "what" your project aims to do? Take the time to focus on the essential elements of the project.

Table 5.1 presents the essential elements of your aims page modeled after the way most senior grantees present their aims. Note that Table 5.1 rather closely conforms to Table 4.1's concept paper elements. If it did not, then it would not lay the necessary tracks to guide a reviewer's *Train of Thought*.

Your research plan strategy pages To re-reiterate, your strategy here is to tell a good story well, not to antagonize the reviewers with surprise twists and distractions. You want to keep them on your *Train of Thought* moving in the direction that you want them to go.

The below list is typical of many NIH RPG application headings. You might wish to use it as a departure point for your section headings where relevant.

1. Background and Significance (Study's contribution to science, practice, policy)
2. Innovation
3. Preliminary Studies/Literature Review
4. Approach/Research Design/Study Protocol

    (a) Aim by aim hypotheses,
    (b) Interventions, data collection and management,
    (c) analysis plan,
    (d) measures,
    (e) participating orgs)

5. Possible Problems (criteria for signaling problems)/Solutions/Limitations,
6. Dissemination and Future Plans
7. Timeline Table of aims by project year
8. Cited References

Given the limited pages applications allow to describe your study, you might expect that applications would be as terse as Wittgenstein's *Tractatus*.[3] Of course, that would be overdoing it, and undermine telling a good story well, as we have recommended.

5.3.3   References/Progress Report

List all cited publications in your research plan – and double check them. One strategy for detecting if you routed your reviewers through some unnecessary side trips or lurches is to review your cited references carefully. If it seems like there are an awful lot, you might have strayed off your strategic train tracks. By examining your references, you might spot one or two that do not seem to logically connect to an aim. Reread the section with the citation to see if you took a side-trip. Removing nonessential verbiage will allow you to make additional points that might help raise reviewer enthusiasm for your project.

Strategically-oriented PIs take the time to examine who sits on relevant IRGs to get a sense of who will most likely review their application. As mentioned earlier, standing IRG/study section rosters of peer reviewers are published on many funding institution websites. That information is important strategically, because if you have a choice of citations, and you only need one or two, picking the one authored by potential reviewers will demonstrate to them that you "really know your science" – if you get our drift. Alternatively, it is always imprudent to denigrate the work of a likely reviewer in justifying your application.

Competing renewals are applications to extend the duration of your project. Publications from your previous grant will weigh heavily on both the peer review panel and during vetting – maybe more so during vetting. If you expect to compete for renewal, it is a good strategy to publish a paper or two that beg the questions you wish to address in the next phase of the project.

5.4   Sample Section

In most cases, federal regulations apply to all research involving humans, animals, or live specimens regardless of whether or not the government is funding the research. If your study involves only **vertebrate animals or live specimens**, there are more details in Sect. 5.4.7. If your study involves **human beings,** unless a study

---

[3] Wittgenstein, L. (1921). Tractatus Logico Philosophicus. *Annalen der Naturphilosophie.*

is Human Subjects Exempt (See Sect. 4.2.4), federal human protection safeguards are mandatory.

If your sample involves humans, and a **medical or behavioral health intervention**, it is a clinical trial. **Clinical trials come with special regulations** over and above other human-involved research (See next section). These special regulations include approval by an Institutional Review Board (IRB – usually convened after a Notice of Grant Award), a *Data and Safety Monitoring Plan (DSMP)*, and if multiple sites are involved, a *Data and Safety Monitoring Board (DSMB)*, and mandatory *Good Clinical Practice Certification* for all key personnel.[4] In addition, close monitoring of enrollment is required to track compliance with mandatory race and gender diversity inclusion as well as the inclusion of children. Thus, requirements outlined in Sects. 5.4.1, 5.4.2, 5.4.3, and 5.4.4 will usually apply to any clinical trial. Appendix B summarizes regulatory compliance issues you might need to address. Finally, all clinical trials must register and enroll with ClinicalTrials.gov.[5]

As mentioned in Sect. 4.2.4, there is a new 2018 consolidated *PHS Human Subjects and Clinical Trials Information* Form in force which helps reduce redundant information previously addressed in research strategy and other application pages. It combines sample descriptions, inclusion criteria, data and safety monitoring, clinical trials, etc. on one web page. Using NIH ASSIST to complete your application helps to ensure compliance.[6]

5.4.1 Protection of Human Subjects

If your study includes human subjects, your application must explain why they must be studied to meet the aims of the proposed research. This is usually straightforward. Describe all the potential risks to subjects posed by participation in the research (physical, psychological, financial, legal, or other), and assess their likelihood and seriousness to the human subjects. Table 5.2 describes essential topics to address in the new human subject protection form.

As the new human subjects form does not have a page limit, be thorough. **The fastest way to fall into the "Not Discussed" category** is to raise a reviewer concern about human subjects protection. While the human subjects protection requirements described here are those associated with NIH, every federal funding institution has similar rules and regulations affecting applications for research involving human subjects. Research that does not conform will have a difficult time being accepted by the Food and Drug Administration (FDA). Federal FOAs will contain links to the relevant protection protocols and required information and assurances for grant applicants.

---

[4] See https://grants.nih.gov/sites/default/files/Clinical-Trials-Changes-full%20length_v5.pptx for more details.

[5] See https://grants.nih.gov/policy/clinical-trials/reporting/index.htm for details.

[6] Go to https://public.era.nih.gov/assist to enroll in NIH ASSIST.

Table 5.2 Major human subjects protection topics	1. Recruitment practices (informed consent, anonymity)
	2. Risks to subjects
	3. Protections against risks (data and safety monitoring)
	4. Benefits of participation
	5. Benefits to science and practice

How do you know if your study is a clinical trial? The categorization has become complex, but NIH breaks clinical trials down to four categories. The Phase III clinical trial category has the most strings tied to safeguard reports and ongoing monitoring to maximize patient safety because often investigators intend to seek FDA approval.

Phase I. Tests a new **biomedical** intervention in a <u>small group</u> of people (e.g. 20–80) for the first time to determine efficacy and evaluate safety (e.g., determine a safe dosage range and identify side effects).

Phase II. Study the **biomedical or behavioral** intervention in a <u>larger group</u> of people, and may include a no-treatment, alternative treatment control groups, and groups with different dosage levels to determine efficacy and further evaluate safety.

Phase III. Study to <u>determine efficacy</u> of the **biomedical or behavioral** intervention in large groups of people (from several hundred to several thousand) by **comparing the intervention to other standard or experimental interventions** as well as to monitor adverse effects, and to collect information that will allow the interventions to be used safely.

Phase IV. Studies conducted after the intervention has been marketed. These studies are designed to <u>monitor the effectiveness</u> of the approved intervention in the general population and to collect information about any adverse effects associated with widespread use.

Regardless of the funding institution type, the awardee institution **must maintain a valid Federal-wide Assurance (FWA) with the NIH Office of Human Research Protections** and obtain approval of the study protocol annually through you IRB to ensure subject privacy and safety. Regulations have been interpreted in such a way that virtually all studies involving humans fall under protection requirements – exemptions are very rare. Appendix B provides more details.

5.4.2 Data and Safety Monitoring

Data and safety monitoring is mandatory for clinical trials.[7] Nobody wants their IQ score or psychiatric evaluation posted on Facebook. Likewise, nobody wants to be taking a drug that is making other people, possibly themselves, sicker. As mentioned earlier, **A Data and Safety Monitoring Plan (DSMP) is required for all clinical trials regardless of phase.** Although a DSMP is not required for all RPGs involving human subjects, we think it is a good practice to include one. It reassures reviewers that you have a plan of action to avoid disclosure and limit harm related to participation. Protection of data ensures subject privacy. Monitoring data during the project enables spotting trends that might signal increased risk of harm to subjects. In some cases, data may even reflect sufficient symptom increase (bad news) or abatement (good news) to amend a study's protocol. In either situation talk first to your PO, then your IRB and/or Data and Safety Monitoring Board (if you have one).

A Data and Safety Monitoring Board (DSMB) is required for multi-site clinical trials in addition to a single IRB overseeing all sites. When a DSMB is required, the DSMP includes a description of the study as well as the commitment and naming of established scientists who will review trial data as spelled out in each study site's DSMP. The plan is to include periodic reviews of subjects entered into the trial to determine if there are significant differences between the intervention and non-intervention trial groups as well as trial sites to determine if the trial should be stopped or modified due to significant benefits or harm between and within groups (control and intervention).

A DSMP should describe the overall framework for the oversight and monitoring of the study. This should encompass the protocol, phase, intervention(s), target population, subject safety and privacy, risks and benefits involved in the study, data integrity and confidentiality, study coordination, responsibilities and protocols to be followed in event of adverse events.

Any required DSMP should include at least the following five elements:

1. Summary of the Protocol (Interventions, procedures, tests and scans, biospecimen collection, interviews and focus groups, study visits. etc.)

   - Primary and secondary outcome measures/endpoints
   - Sample size and target population
   - Inclusion/exclusion criteria and how the criteria will be evaluated
   - For multi-site trials, a list of proposed participating clinical sites and data coordinating centers and a description of each site's role

2. Roles and Responsibilities (Identification and description of individuals responsible for monitoring the trial their roles, qualifications, and the frequency of all monitoring activities.)
3. Trial Safety:

---

[7] http://grants.nih.gov/grants/guide/notice-files/not98-084.html

- Specific events that would preclude a participant from continuing the intervention
- Procedures in place for managing any medication related issues
- The potential risks and the measures in place to detect them
- The consent/assent procedures (e.g., by whom, how and under what conditions will a subject be consented)
- The mechanisms in place to protect subject privacy
- The trial stopping rules for the study
- The plan for management of incidental findings (e.g., discovering a hidden condition)
- Managing conflicts of interest that may potentially challenge participant safety or bias data)
- For multi-center studies, the monitoring plan for data reporting across study sites
- Data security in place to protect the confidentiality of the data (e.g., encrypted electronic records) and any limits to confidentiality (e.g., suicidal ideation, child abuse)

4. Reportable Events:

- Procedures for documenting and reporting Adverse Events (AEs), Serious Adverse Events (SAEs) , and unanticipated risks.
- Specific plan and timeframe for reporting to the IRB, DSMB, and funding institutions

5. Data Management, Analysis, and Quality Assurance:

- Data sources (e.g., questionnaires, records, biospecimens, recordings)
- Security measures to protect data sources, including how the data will be labeled and stored
- Quality assurance measures for subject recruitment, enrollment, enrollment targets, and for the validity and integrity of the data.

5.4.3 Reporting Adverse Events (AEs)

NIH defines an *Adverse Event (AE)* as any untoward or unfavorable medical occurrence in a human study participant, including any abnormal sign (e.g. abnormal physical exam or laboratory finding), symptom, or disease, temporally associated with the participants' involvement in the research, *whether or not considered related to participation in the research*. For AEs, a written report is due as soon as possible to your IRB and within 15 days to your PO. AEs should also be included in the annual progress report for multi-year awards. AEs often serve as the basis for patent information about the risks and side effects of FDA-approved drugs and other interventions.

A *Serious Adverse Event (SAE)* occurs when, if, in the view of either the PI or the study sponsor, *an adverse event results in death, is life-threatening, requires inpatient hospitalization, prolongs an existing hospitalization, results in (a) a persistent or significant incapacity or substantial disruption of the ability to conduct normal life functions, (b) a congenital anomaly/birth defect, or (c) some medical intervention is required to prevent any of these AEs.* Any SAE should be reported to your PO immediately via phone or email even before alerting the IRB and DSMB. Prompt PO notification allows the funding institution ample time to prepare for possible press and Congressional inquiries. A written SAE report to the IRB and PO is due within 7 days.

5.4.4   Inclusion of Women and Minorities

Review panels will also assess the adequacy of plans to include subjects from both genders, all racial and ethnic groups (and subgroups), and children, as appropriate, for the scientific goals of the research. Plans for the recruitment and retention of subjects will also be evaluated. See Scott (2004) for tips on improving the retention of human subjects.

5.4.5   Inclusion of Children

If you are <u>not</u> including children (defined by NIH as anyone under age 18), you must explain why not. There are many sound reasons for sample restriction, but most common is that children are not affected by whatever it is you are studying, (e.g., adult-onset diabetes, Alzheimer's disease, shingles). If you include children, you must describe their characteristics.

5.4.6   Target/Planned Enrollment Table

You might say that you are going to include women and minorities, the sample enrollment table excerpted from PHS Form 398 in Fig. 5.2 (or something similar) is how you demonstrate your adherence to that plan. NIH requires that the table be updated at least annually to enable POs to monitor progress. Difficulty adhering to the Enrollment Table is one of the most common reasons RPGs go into no-cost extensions.

5.4.7   Vertebrate Animals

If you are planning to use live vertebrate animals in the project, you must adhere to the requirements in the Public Health Service (PHS) Policy on Humane Care and Use of Laboratory Animals whether or not NIH is your funding institution.[8] In case

---

[8] https://grants.nih.gov/grants/olaw/references/phspolicylabanimals.pdf provides details.

Program Director/Principal Investigator (Last, First, Middle):

Targeted/Planned Enrollment Table

This report format should NOT be used for data collection from study participants.

Study Title:

Total Planned Enrollment:

TARGETED/PLANNED ENROLLMENT: Number of Subjects			
Ethnic Category	Females	Males	Total
Hispanic or Latino			
Not Hispanic or Latino			
Ethnic Category: Total of All Subjects *			
Racial Categories			
American Indian/Alaska Native			
Asian			
Native Hawaiian or Other Pacific Islander			
Black or African American			
White			
Racial Categories: Total of All Subjects *			

* The "Ethnic Category: Total of All Subjects" must be equal to the "Racial Categories: Total of All Subjects."

Fig. 5.2   Typical NIH Targeted/Planned Enrollment Table (from PHS398)

you were wondering, yes there are AE and SAE reporting requirements for animals too. If you think about it, any contamination to animal subjects risks invalidating the study. In the case of disease, then entire population in the vivarium might be as risk of expiration, not to mention human caretakers!

5.4.8   Select Agents

It is quite rare that a new investigator will be using select agents. Briefly, select agents are hazardous biological agents and toxins that HHS or USDA have identified as having the potential to pose a severe threat to public health and safety, to animal and plant health, or to animal and plant products. CDC maintains a list of HHS and USDA Select Agents and Toxins at www.selectagents.gov . If you are using select agents you must describe methods for obtaining them, ensuring safety in shipment, ensuring a secure and appropriate method of storage during your study, safety measures on site such as first aid kits and eyewash stations, protective clothing to be worn, who will have access and under what condition, and, describe measures to minimize any foreseeable risks to human or animal subjects.

5.5   Collaboration

As we have reiterated, science is a collaborative endeavor. Even the fictional Dr. Frankenstein had Igor. Normally, collaboration is a good thing in a grant application. This is especially the case for new investigators. Adding senior investigators as Co-Is or consultants can markedly help reduce the perceived risk of not achieving project aims. New investigators should avoid using a Co-PI because NIH does not recognize that status as "independent." To NIH, Co-PI is just another Co-I.

5.5.1   Leadership

Generally speaking, being a principal investigator means you are responsible for navigating the grant application process and seeing the project through to completion and possibly a competing renewal. Whether or not you took a course in management or leadership in college, as a PI you will have to both manage and lead to be successful. You are the face of the project to the funding organization and the public. You are also responsible for marketing your project both prior to receiving a grant, and during the life of the grant. It will be your publications that justify to peers and funding agencies that your project is a good investment. You will be the project's motivating force whether deciding to revise and resubmit, persisting in the face of unforeseen barriers, or changing course when events and results demand. Submission of a leadership plan is mandatory for complex projects in which there are multiple PIs – unlikely if you are just starting out.

All PIs are created equal in the eyes of NIH, and all PIs are equally responsible for conduct of their projects. As a new investigator, you might join a study as a **Co-PI** in the leadership plan, but that **designation holds no special status with NIH officials** – just the other project investigators. Projects you might join include Multi-Headed R01s and Multi-Headed Cooperative projects (U01/P01).

The Multi-Headed R01 The R01 is an individual grant award, however, you may have **one or more Co-PIs/Co-Is** (both roles are equivalent). The applicant institution is responsible for deciding the number of PIs on individual grant awards. **NIH only recognizes one PI per grant.**

The Multi-Headed Cooperative (U01/P01) Described in Chap. 2 as large grants, Cooperative and Center grants normally involve pooling data from multiple studies, multiple PIs and multiple sites. Although large grants are uncommon, as a new investigator you might find yourself in the role of Co-PI/I on a multi-PI grant. U01s differ from P01s in that U01 s normally involve multiple institutions, whereas PO1s are normally located a one institution. The exception is the UM1 or UM2. They involve multiple centers as discussed as an Extra-Large grant in Chap. 2.

Clearly multi-headed projects create a Hydra of a dragon which is unlikely to work smoothly unless there is a leadership plan that makes sense. Thus, serious discussion among investigators before drafting the plan will help to reassure reviewers that good communication and cooperation among investigators is likely. Our experience as a science officers on several cooperative projects suggests that the most-respected PI, regardless of academic rank, usually has the best success as PI of record as long as that person has a bit of charm and charisma.

5.5.2 Consortium/Contractual Agreements

It may be necessary to collaborate with a Co-I from a different organization/institution from yours. The nature of the arrangement between the grantee institution and the collaborating institution is addressed in this section of the application. For smaller grants, consortium agreements are often necessary when contracting out parts of the research program. Those agreements should go into the application appendices.

5.5.3 Letters of Support (LOS)

The more up-front support for your project that you can demonstrate in the application, the less risky your project will appear. As mentioned in the previous chapter, not demonstrating support for things like subject access, essential equipment, and service resources will often add to the apparent risk of your project. Thus, a good LOS details the specifics of what the signed is agreeing to. You also want enthusiastic LOSs from key personnel on the project. Letters of support are normally included in your application appendix.

5.5.4 Resource Sharing Plan

If you are advancing science, then sharing with your colleagues nicely demonstrates your commitment. If you have an NIH grant, and you are receiving more than **$500 K** in any grant year, or if your research involves a genome-wide association study (**GWAS**) you MUST include a data and/or resource sharing plan. If yours is a clinical trial, ClinicalTrials.gov is your sharing resource. There are three categories for sharing plans: (a) data sharing, (b) model organisms, and (c) genomic data. The FOA will indicate which plan(s) are required. The most common is the **Data Sharing Plan (DSP)** . In that plan you should include conference presentations, updates in newsletters, a blog site open to colleagues and/or the public, contribution of your data (at what point in time) to a data archive that supports secondary data analysis, and the like. You should also include methods for protecting confidentiality such as stripping data of identifying names, demographics, or other information that might single them out in secondary analysis.

You may include a DSP even if it does not involve a GWAS or cost over half a million dollars. A DSP will often engender enthusiasm among both peer and funding institution reviewers. **Data & Resource Sharing Plan (DRSP)** guidance and examples are provided online.[9]

5.5.5 *Authentication of Biological/Chemical Resources*

Research performed with unreliable or misidentified resources can negate years of hard work and eliminate any chance for a study to be reproduced or expanded upon. Thus, it is imperative that you describe methods you will use to ensure the identity and validity of key biological and/or chemical resources used in your project. Generally speaking, standard laboratory reagents that are not expected to vary do not need to be included in the plan. Examples are buffers and other common biologicals or chemicals.

5.6 Application Appendices

This is where you put all the other stuff you could not fit into your research plan that you HOPE reviewers will examine and be thrilled to see, or at least impressed. **Keep in mind that there is no requirement for reviewers to examine appendices**, but most do. Principal reviewers usually will examine appended material if it clarifies something. In practice, reviewers often examine the credibility of letters of support, experimental or new survey measures, interview protocols, etc.

If you try to use appendices as a means to increase your application story, that strategy is as precarious and the cowboy trying to jump from his horse onto your speeding *Train of Thought*. You might get your application returned unscored. Only include materials not readily available elsewhere, as well as complicated algorithms or lengthy complex derivations when their content is critical to hypothesis tests.

A good rule of thumb is to put yourself in the reviewer's position. If you were reviewing your application, would you want to see: a mathematical proof? the items in the questionnaire? a two-sentence LOS with no details about what is being committed to? your consent forms? et cetera? If the answer is something like "Not very likely." Then it is probably best to leave it out.

---

[9] https://grants.nih.gov/grants/policy/data_sharing/data_sharing_guidance.htm   and   at   https://grants.nih.gov/policy/sharing.htm

Keep in mind that your goal is to convince reviewers that your project is solid science technically, contributes to scientific theory, and advances the funding institution's mission. Excessive detail always runs the risk of creating distractions and questions being raised about methods that may have little bearing on the overall technical merit of the project. Nevertheless, if your details led reviewers to raise questions regarding your approach, guess what else is likely to rise – your score?

Chapter 6
Application Review

Application Review

- Assign to Agency/Inst.
- Assign Prog. Official
- Assign to Review Panel
- Conduct Peer Review

Once your application for a grant or contract has been formally accepted by the funding institution, it goes into their scientific review and vetting cycles. We make a distinction here between peer review by an IRG for *technical merit* (Initial Review), and *funding institution/agency vetting for prioritizing awards* (Secondary Review). You gain a strategic advantage when drafting a grant application if you understand the process of how it will be evaluated. Thus, this chapter offers considerable grantsmanship insight.

At NIH, scientific review and vetting are firewalled within the institution. This enables program staff to play an active role in administering the programs of research under their cognizance. Firewalling also allows POs the freedom to help applicants maximize project-mission fit with the IC when crafting their applications. Not all agencies bar program administrators from participating in review. The National Science Foundation (NSF) is a good example. NSF does not involve their advisory councils/boards in discrete grant funding decisions. After peer review, it is normally up to the discretion of program officials to make award decisions based upon technical merit alone because NSF's focus is on basic science. Conversely, most other federal agencies need to tie funding decisions to mission goals.

6.1 Assignment to Agency/Institution

Using NIH as an example, once your application arrives in the Grants.Gov system directly or via ASSIST, the "Initial Review" stage begins. The agency office responsible for managing applications (in NIH's case the Center for Scientific Review – CSR) first reviews the application for completeness and responsiveness. Your

© The Author(s), under exclusive license to Springer Nature Switzerland AG 2019   77
T. F. Hilton, C. G. Leukefeld, *Grantsmanship for New Investigators*,
SpringerBriefs in Public Health, https://doi.org/10.1007/978-3-030-01301-1_6

application goes to both the CSR (or similar arm of other funding institutions) for assignment to a peer review panel and to an NIH Institute or Center (IC) for administration. Once assigned to an IC, your application is further assigned to a division within the IC for assignment to a branch, which assigns it to a specific program official (PO), who shepherds your application through review and vetting, and who, as we have explained earlier, becomes your project officer (also PO) if your grant is awarded.

Usually institute and subsequent division, branch, and PO assignment is straightforward because many FOAs are IC and PO-specific. Generic BAAs/FOAs that have multiple IC sponsorship (meaning you may apply to any of them) require you to choose an IC. If you think your application was assigned to the wrong IC, division, branch, PO, or IRG, call your assigned PO. They can usually get your application reassigned or explain to you why what appears to be a misassignment is in fact appropriate. In many cases, when assigned POs recognize a mistake they will request reassignment to a more appropriate PO on the spot.

6.2 Assignment to a Review Panel

Once your application has been deemed to be a good fit with NIH IC requirements, and all paperwork appears to be complete, a Scientific Review Officer (SRO) is assigned to oversee its peer review. The SRO, in turn, assigns the application to an IRG with the necessary expertise to review the application and will designate several IRG members as principal reviewers – usually three – to provide written critiques. The entire IRG sees your application and each member assigns a score once the principal reviewers have each described the project and offered their scored opinion of its technical merit, following the criteria previously overviewed in Table 1.2.

Which NIH IRG gets an application for peer review is normally decided by CSR based on the FOA against which you are applying, the types of expertise required to adequately determine technical merit, and the expertise you requested on the PHS Assignment Request Form (PHS ARF). How can you minimize misassignments? As we have mentioned, it pays to get familiar with the members of the review panel likely to review your application. If confused about which IRG is best, email your PO. They will normally be able to point you in the optimal direction. IRG standing members are listed on nearly all agency websites.

Keep in mind, that most reviewers are senior people who often serve on journal editorial boards and have reviewed dozens if not hundreds of grant applications. If you present your application story well, most reviewers, regardless of project-related expertise, can determine if your project is well-designed and appropriate to the funding institution's mission. If the review panel chair thinks the application is not appropriate, the IRG/study section chair will inform CSR and request assignment for review elsewhere.

6.3   The Review Process

The application review process is like a rollercoaster. It is by far the one aspect of the grant application experience that is the most mysterious and anxiety-provoking to applicants – new and senior. It is also one of the most complex in the context of the entire vetting process, of which peer review is only one stage – albeit a critical one. Every applicant understands the process from their personal experience colored by theories and observations shared by colleagues. A contributing factor that helps to create distortion is that having your work judged by your peers is an emotionally-charged experience. There is so much riding on the outcome, and everybody in your organization knows you are applying. Thus, not getting funded risks some loss of face.

Another contributing factor to distorted perceptions of peer review is that funding agencies often use diverse models to review applications. They may use video teleconferences, face-to-face meetings in Washington, emails, and on-line chat sessions; and they may combine several of these approaches – especially if a special ad hoc reviewer is needed for only one or two applications. Often the review format is related to the funding mechanism. Large grants are more likely to enjoy face-to-face meetings than are smaller grants. Agencies regularly tinker with the review process as new technology evolves as reviews are expensive. Thus, perceptions of the process are often colored by your luck of the draw.

Having sat in on many reviews in many formats, we are both impressed by how fairly reviews proceed regardless of format. The modality of review appears to have little impact on the validity of the reviews. Nevertheless, some modalities minimize or even obviate the give-and-take among the entire panel during reviews. It is more difficult to detect sarcasm and humor using only audio communication or chat than it is video telecons and face-to-face meetings. That is one reason NIH uses face-to-face meetings to vet larger grant applications. Training grants and special and irregular mechanisms that involve low-complexity applications are more likely to rely on less costly, less time-consuming review modalities.

6.4   Assignment to Program Official (PO)/Director

As we touched on in Sect. 1.4, once a project is funded, your assigned PO/PD oversees administration of the research for the life of the grant in the role of *Project Officer*. There is only one PO per grant, but that PO might have a steering committee of POs for some Extra-Large RPGs involving multiple ICs.

Finally, there is a second federal research official who can pop up. This is the Science Officer (SO). SOs are usually assigned to any project in which the Federal Government has a significant stake in the outcome, project sensitivity requires a presence in the laboratory, or a project is highly complex involving multiple institutions and PIs. SOs are considered co-investigators (Co-I's) by the funding agency because they work intimately with the research team. SOs may be authors on project publications. The primary role of the SO is to monitor day-to-day decisions, and ensure effective execution of the project, progress in achieving project aims, and effective coordination with other project institutions. SOs report to both the PI and the PO, and they may sit on both project and agency steering committees for multi-institution projects and cooperatives. As experienced researchers knowledgeable about government regulations, like ambassadors, SOs are best equipped to justify or explain to the PO any problems, proposed changes, or deviations from the project plan. Although it might seem that SOs are agency spies, they are assigned to help ensure a project's success; not to undermine it. At NIH, most SOs involved in extramural grant research are POs who are assigned as a collateral duty. SOs may not serve as in a dual capacity as PO on the same project.

If you have been in contact with a funding institution PO prior to submission, it is prudent to alert them once your application has been submitted. When Tom got such calls, he would alert division and his branch chief that a project he encouraged was in the system. Alerts help to ensure that branch chiefs assign projects to a PO with interest in the application. In most cases, identifying the relevant PO is obvious.

There may be times when an application is assigned to a PO other than the one with whom you have been in contact. It might be because the RFA to which you are responding belongs to a different PO's portfolio. If it is due to administrative misassignments, the PO with whom you worked can arrange for reassignment. However, if the PO thinks that your application will do better in another institute, division, or branch PO's portfolio, they will let you know. Program direction is a team effort. POs are not in competition with one another. They do not get bonuses in their paycheck for the number of grants in their portfolios.

6.5 Review Meetings

Scientific Review Officers (SROs) are nearly always mid or late career PhDs familiar with their field. Their job is to first validate that they are the correct person to be responsible for the review of your application. If not, they will transfer it to a more appropriate SRO. Their goal is an unbiased review. The SRO determines the review format. As mentioned already, large applications are usually reviewed face-to-face in the Washington, DC area by IRGs meeting in meeting rooms near where the reviewers are staying. Sometimes, review panels meet on the West Coast to reduce travel costs and accommodate IRGs with a large number of members west of the Mississippi or sometimes right after professional conferences in the city where they were held. POs usually may monitor via video telecon if they cannot travel.

When POs sit in on reviews, they get a better sense of the discussion than can be gleaned from your written post-review summary sheet critiques. **POs are free to share their impressions of the review with applicants, and to advocate for their assigned projects during vetting**. Keep in mind that your PO may not be able to attend every review due to schedule conflicts. Nevertheless, POs do try to attend as many as possible.

6.6   Scoring

Grant organizations put a lot of store in peer review scores, and they should. If you do not score low enough, the odds of funding are rather dismal. However, as we discuss in Chap. 7, even if your application scores in a competitive range, there is no guarantee of funding.

Table 1.2 in Chap. 1 lists the seven major review criteria used by NIH and most funding agencies. NIH uses a formal scoring system, which is **like a handicapping system**. The higher the score; the less competitive the application. Although the final IRG impact score can run from 10 to 90, IRGs only score applications primary reviewers nominate to be in the top 50% of those reviewed. Thus, fewer than half usually score below 50. Applications judged to be in the bottom 50% are normally "Not Discussed (ND)" and go unscored – out of competition.

Not Discussed (ND) Applications are nominated at the beginning of the review meeting by the primary reviewers as being in the bottom half of the submissions for the review meeting. The reviewers briefly explain their concerns, and the entire IRG panel votes not to discuss the application. **The decision not to discuss must be unanimous.** If one or more reviewer requests that an application be scored, then it is reviewed. Otherwise, the two or three primary reviewers document weaknesses and strengths in the written summary statement that all applicants receive. These weaknesses help applicants judge whether to revise the application and try for a second review. Probably 9 out of 10 times, when an ND-nominated application is discussed, it winds up being scored above 50 anyway, and is voted ND. This usually happens when a reviewer is enthusiastic about the project question and overlooks a serious weakness that arises early in the subsequent discussion.

IRG Panel Review Procedures
1. Primary Reviewers. The primary reviewers assigned to each application usually consists of a primary, secondary, and third or fourth reviewer. Each prepare written reviews which are posted on the secure meeting website as review summary statements. Strengths and weaknesses are bulleted for each review criteria. These same reviewers score each review criteria, and give an overall impact score using a range of 1–9 for each of the five criteria listed Table 1.2.
2. Presentation. Primary reviewers first nominate applications to be not discussed or scored. A unanimous concurrence by the IRG results in no score or discussion, and applicants only receive written feedback explaining weaknesses. Primary reviewers then present the aims for each remaining top 50% application to the review panel and point out perceived strengths and weaknesses along with their preliminary impact score. Reviewers are usually selected for project-specific expertise. Remaining primary reviewers make complementary remarks and offer their preliminary impact scores.
3. Discussion of Budget & Human/Animal Concerns. The entire IRG panel then discuss the application's technical merit, before addressing criteria 6 – Human & Animal subjects treatment and criteria 7 – budget appropriateness. Usually,

major concerns, will move a score into the unfundable range. If concerns are egregious, a rare occasion, the application may receive a vote that it is not recommended for further consideration (**NRFC**). That means NIH will not consider a revised submission. Finally, they discuss criteria 7, and mention if budget elements seem reasonable. They may recommend cuts or increases.

4. Voting. Following discussion, each member of the IRG panel votes a score of 1–9 within the range established by the highest and lowest primary reviewer scores (e.g., between 1 and 3). Those scores are then averaged by the SRO and multiplied times 10 to create a final panel-voted impact score ranging from 10 to 90. They are later percentiled for perspective. An IRG member may vote outside the recommended range, but must justify their vote (high or low) in writing, which is added to the applicant's summary statement. The SRO edits and distributes the official summary statement, and they may include comments from other review panel members that might help highlight concerns.

6.6.1 POs and Review

Before discussing the review process, it seems appropriate to discuss the role of your PO in the process both before, during, and after applications are scored. Why listen to advice from some Washington bureaucrat? Keep in mind that most POs likely listen to several a hundred grant reviews each year. That is far more review exposure than one could accrue serving on a standing peer review panel for many years. Another reason to heed their advice is that they know the institution to which you are applying inside and out. Thus, that knowledge can help you navigate the bureaucracy when you get lost in it. Finally, the majority of POs are seasoned veteran researchers who joined the government from a variety of academic and research settings. For many, they gave up tenured positions because their spouse relocated to the DC Metro area or they were recruited by NIH staff. When Tom joined NIH, two thirds of his branch at NIDA were over age 50. Most had held academic appointments, worked as bench and community researchers, and like Carl and Tom, had managed large projects, and led laboratories and clinics.

6.6.2 What If You Get a Low Score?

If you get a score below 2.5, you are likely to get an award. As you score increases, the odds of deferral or not getting on the IC's Funding Plan increases, and you will have to decide to wait to see if you get funded, elect to revise and resubmit in hopes of getting a more competitive score, or as the majority of new applicants do – just walk away. In that last case, you might want to start reconsidering your future career as a researcher.

6.6.3   What If You Get a Low Score, But Funding Is Deferred?

Deferral decisions are almost always for funding institution/agency budgetary reasons. Even though your project has been judged to have technical merit, that is not the only factor in play when making funding decisions. The following are our suggests for what you can do to move your project on a fundable trajectory.

1. Marketing: You can help the funding institution identify willing co-funding institutions by marketing your application and summary statement to other institutes or agencies as well as private foundations. [Talk to your PO to avoid working at cross purposes.]
2. Self-Funding: You might get your dean to absorb more project costs by donating equipment or space that would lower the cost of your project.
3. Surgery: You might propose to delete a hypothesis or project arm to lower project costs without reducing its perceived value of the project overall. Think *level of effort* here. Modifying the scope of your project is a particularly helpful strategy if your summary statement questions one arm of your study. For example, by eliminating one intervention group or control group, you could reduce costs significantly, but still be viewed by the funding institution as having a worthwhile project. You might eliminate a costly assay or other measure that addressed a potential moderator variable. In any case, discuss design changes you are willing to make with your PO to get their opinion as to whether or not such post-score changes will improve a revised submission, or possibly help them promote funding your project without a resubmission.
4. Waiting: It might just be that your project was submitted with a large number of outstanding projects or your project was relatively expensive. Therefore, NIH institutes will often wait one or two funding cycles to see if the next applications are less competitive or less costly than yours. Those residual funds might add up to your grant award.
5. Revise and Resubmit: Finally, you can redesign your study and/or decrease costs while keeping the science intact in the hope that a second review will shave off more points from your score. You and your funding institution have your summary statement to inform your next step. If scored low but deferred, you already know that your idea is meritorious. You often just need to lower costs or tighten up your design (confirm that with your PO). Strategically, if revision can be done within several weeks, you might be able to resubmit in time for the next review cycle. Why would you decide to do that? Because strategically, you have two studies in the queue. If the initial application is funded before your revised application is scored, you can withdraw your revised application without any consequence. If the first application is not picked up during the next cycle, you already have a more competitive alternative application in review.

Paylines   Some funding institutions use fixed percentiles or scores to establish a "payline" or "funding line" above which a scored project will NOT usually be funded. Paylines are merely advisory to help applicants decide if they need to start thinking about a revise and resubmit scenario even before getting their summary statements. Always ask your PO for their take on your funding potential.

6.6.4   What If You Get a High Score?

Getting a high score is in most cases similar to being non-scored. So why do review panels give high scores? When you receive a score between 28 and 35, it gives the IC the option of deferring a funding decision to see if funds become available. Some minor flaws are straightforwardly fixable without a resubmission, and might be worked out with your PO if there is high enthusiasm for the project. Regardless, you always have the option to revise to see if you can get a lower score. In most cases when an applicant receives a score above 35, it indicates that some IRG panel members considered some concerns to be more onerous than other members did. As the score increases, so also are the number of issues that must be addressed. Of course, you have more than scores to guide your next move. You have the summary statement and your PO's impression.

6.6.5   What If You Want to Appeal Your Score?

It doesn't happen often, but sometimes applicants feel strongly that they have been unfairly reviewed. Appeals are rare, and successful appeals are rarer yet. The most common reaction of a funding institution is to request a few additional ad hoc reviews. It has been our experience that additional reviews seldom result in substantial changes in competitiveness. Appeals could delay your application revision by shortening the time available for you to see your new score and summary statement in time revise and resubmit before the next application deadline. **If additional reviews are unlikely to change the score enough to merit funding, then there is little point in appealing** – painful as that may be to your ego. That is why your PO is the best person with whom to brainstorm. If your PO encourages an appeal, then you might benefit from additional reviews. Every case is unique.

Conflict of Interest If you believe that an IRG member has a conflict of interest related to your project notify the SRO prior to the review meeting. Normal practice is to ask panel members to recuse themselves from the reviews in which they have conflicts. Conflicted reviewers leave the room until scoring of the conflict application is complete. In addition, if potential conflict or bias is identified before the summary score is released, SROs may delete a reviewer's score, and edit or redact their comments from the summary statement. However, because there may be 20 or more other reviewers on the panel, deleting an N of 1 is unlikely to appreciably change your score. If your PO attended, she or he can offer their impression of the impact a conflicted reviewer may have had on the rest of the panel.

Incorrect or Unfair Criticism Sometimes reviewers get it wrong or cite a criticized or retracted study when justifying a concern. The first reaction of some applicants is; "Gotcha!" However, when applicants believed they got an unfair review, POs can often point to other weaknesses mentioned in summary statements that <u>are</u> valid and sufficiently problematic to justify an unfundable or high score. Thus, you might be right, but you still need to revise and resubmit.

Unfamiliar Methods or Technology As mentioned earlier, a few times we supported appeals because we believed that the reviewers demonstrated an insufficient grasp of the methods or technology in the application. This can happen when projects plow new scientific turf or employ cutting-edge methods. When this occurs, summary statements and meeting remarks often betray unfamiliarity with the proposed project. In the rare instances in which this happened during our tenure, the SROs concurred with our perception, and arranged for special reviews. If the score was relatively low, we could sometimes argue for funding without additional review. Again, this sort of situation is quite rare.

6.6.6 What If You Are Unscored/Not Discussed?

When an application is not discussed (ND) by the review committee, you have to either abandon the project or revise and resubmit your application. Carl's personal experience as a PI has been that getting an ND is emotionally deflating. Rejection rocks our self-esteem and leads most people to feel heightened negative emotions. Neuroscience has demonstrated that there is a negative correlation between emotion and cognition (Mather and Fanselow 2018; Okon-Singer 2018). The more upset we are; the less clearly we are likely to reason. That is why **we recommend holding off on any action or reaction** (besides disappointment) **until seeing your summary statement and subsequently talking things over with your PO**. It might take a month or more after scores are released depending on the SRO's schedule. Almost always peer criticism is motivated by the desire to be helpful.

Often an ounce of PO encouragement is worth a pound of your enthusiasm to revise. When working in the role of PO, Carl and Tom regularly encountered applicants who were surprised by our encouragement to revise. "What? I got a 49!"

Upset, many applicants overlook important criticisms while exaggerating the importance of minor ones. Most problems that undermine a competitive score can be fixed. That is when POs and mentors can help you put your application's strengths and weaknesses into more realistic perspective. Peer criticism is rarely scolding. When it is, it is usually because you violated safety norms, or some other regulation. You might have a rare unfixable application. However, in most cases, future success usually hinges on making improvements, and then resubmitting your revised application.

You may revise and resubmit an NIH application an infinite number of times. If a revised submission fails to get funded, applicants may re-apply yet again, but it will be treated as a new application. The effect of that change is that SROs try to have the same primary reviewers score your revision. In addition, revisions get an extra page to respond to reviews – new (3rd) applications do not. The second revision might be seen by new primary reviewers, and you lose out on telling your IRG panel what you fixed. If the third time is not the proverbial charm, then perhaps the adage "Three strikes and you're out." bears consideration.

6.6.7   How Do You Revise an Application?

There are quite a few things that applicants can do to improve their resubmission. Here are four of the most common fixes.

Fixing Errors of Omission Inexperience, page limits, or haste normally cause investigators to inadvertently omit some key information. Applications are notoriously complicated, and inexperience can lead to oversights. When that happens, reviewers usually include encouraging language such as: "Additional details about the confidential handling of patient information would strengthen the application." Nevertheless, even when you receive encouraging feedback, you should re-review every word in your application to ensure that you made your best case. Why? Because sometimes, **when you clarify one thing, it can raise an entirely new set of concerns about something else, and/or confirm that the panel's concerns were justified**.

Fixing Errors of Commission This is re-addressed here in the context of how committing an error can lead to being unscored. Usually errors of commission are from a lack of balanced procedural descriptions. If your narrative gets too deep into the weeds in one section, you risk raising questions about inadequately-described procedures elsewhere in the application. Simply put, when you say you are going to do something in section "A" but fail to adequately describe a related action in section "B" or "C", you inadvertently set yourself up for criticism.

Assuaging Concerns About Expertise In most cases, expertise concerns can be blunted by adding one or two consultants to the team, or by increasing the time commitment of certain team members. Summary statements usually indicate the nexus of expertise concerns.

Dispelling Human & Animal Subjects Concerns Human subjects (HS) concerns are a common reason applications have historically gone unscored or got high, unfundable scores. With the 2018 revision of the SF 424, Human and Animal Subjects no longer compete for space in the in the application research plan as there is a separate section for that now, and for example, during recruitment – were patients assured that not volunteering would have no (zero) impact on their continued treatment? Did the PI adequately describe procedures to assure that recruitment and data management will be conducted in a way that protects privacy and ensures adverse effects will be noticed in time to safely intervene? Will procedures enable the correct consolidation of various measurements with the correct case? [Yes, these kinds of oversights have rendered large RPGs to receive unfundable scores.] Similarly, failure to justify the use of animals, to inadequately describe humane treatment, or to ensure animal care post-study can lead to unfundable applications. Lastly, if using select agents, failure to safeguard them from public exposure risks causing a pandemic. So, you can imagine that procedures must be – might we say – air-tight. We encourage using checklists to help ensure that adequate assurances are addressed in your application.

6.7 Other Government Review Processes

This section address differences for several other Federal funding institutions review processes. Some are not always as involved as NIH in human subjects research. Thus, life and death issues might be relatively less common. Moreover, technical merit review might be more or less challenging than at NIH, whereas vetting for budgets and mission-fit might be more detailed and demanding than NIH.

6.7.1 The Department of Defense (DOD)

DOD grants and contracts should be pursued by individuals who are familiar with DOD research and development. Not only is familiarity with the mission, operations, and regulations of the targeted Service (Army, Navy (includes the Marine Corps), Air Force) usually essential, but also too is having appropriate security clearances. Clearances can take many months to obtain, and a catch-22 is that they are issued on a need-to-know basis. Thus, the most straightforward way to get a clearance is to work on somebody's classified project before applying on your own.

DOD Review panels are normally composed of senior DOD intramural researchers augmented by outside ad hoc scientists. Not unlike NIH, multi-million/multi-year grants and contracts at DOD are often reviewed first by extramural scientists to determine technical merit. A second stage might include an intramural review panel to ensure alignment and budget issues are a good fit. Finally, funding priorities are decided by Service-specific stake holders to determine mission requirement fit – not unlike NIH's procedures. Contrary to popular belief, the lowest bidder does not always get the contract or grant. As with all extramural federal research, vetting includes getting "the best bang for the buck."

Grants Most Department of Defense extramural research is done via contracts; not grants. There are exceptions. Most notably are the Defense Advanced Research Project Agency (DARPA) grants. DARPA projects are usually large, and awarded to established universities and institutions, which have an established relationship with DOD. FOAs for Armed Services grants are published in Broad Agency Announcements (BAAs) on **Grants.Gov.**

Contracts Each military service has intramural research capabilities, so research contracts are most often used to augment expertise or capabilities not available in-house. Contract FOAs are announced on **FedBizOps.gov** (use https://www.fbo.gov). Nearly all federal agencies, NIH as well, use Requests For Proposals (**RFPs**) to meet emergent or high-priority contract needs. Like grant RFAs, contract RFPs often have defined budget ceilings and short time frames to apply.

6.7.2 Department of Veterans Affairs (VA)

All Veterans Affairs research is intramural. Although the VA publishes FOAs similar to the NIH, only in-house VA researchers may apply for funding. If you are on a campus with a VA Medical Center, you might be able join a VA research project if invited. Many VA researchers have or pursue joint appointments with medical schools to conduct research. Thus, the VA is having its intramural cake and eating its extramural cake too. The VA can also solicit contract work on **FedBizOps.gov** to tap technical expertise in areas such as prosthetics and surgical instruments. If you are on a campus with VA ties, find out who is working in your area and explore collaboration. It might lead to more than a joint appointment.

6.7.3 National Science Foundation (NSF)

The US National Science Foundation was established by Congress in 1950 "To promote the progress of science; to advance the national health, prosperity, and welfare; and to secure the national defense." (Gonzales 2014). Despite its wide charter, NSF's emphasis (as amended over the years) is on basic science research across all areas of science except those funded by other agencies. Thus, for example, health science is the exclusive purview of NIH, aerospace belongs to NASA, etc. Because NSF grants are generally not applied but are basic science projects, funding priorities are less influenced by Legislative and Executive branch priorities; and as mentioned earlier, mission-fit is rarely a review issue.

With an annual budget of roughly $7BN, NSF funds about a quarter of all university-based basic science research. FOAs are posted on Grants.Gov. Similar to NIH, NSF supports training and career development grants. As we mentioned earlier, NSF POs are more directly involved in award decisions than are NIH POs. As such, NSF POs are more limited in what information they can offer to guide application development than POs at NIH. NSF advice to applicants is normally limited to clarifying FOA content and providing general information on the application and review process.

The NSF review process is similar to NIH and relies upon extramural peer review panels to judge applications technical merit. However, at NSF the higher the score the better. NSF scores range from 1 to 5 with 5 being excellent (the opposite of NIH). Vetting decisions are somewhat different from NIH in that mission interface and government priorities rarely play a role. The NSF vetting process results in awards to about 1 out of 5 applications – similar to the award rate at NIH (von Hippel and von Hippel, 2015).

6.7.4 National Aeronautics and Space Administration (NASA)

NASA funds intramural and extramural research primarily through solicited proposals for grants (see Grants.Gov), and relies upon cooperative agreements, contracts and arrangements with other agencies, non-profit organizations, industry and academia. Solicitation mechanisms primarily used are NASA Research Announcements (NRAs), Announcements of Opportunity (AOs), and Cooperative Agreement Notices (CANs). A few unsolicited proposals are also considered.

NASA invests on the order of $3 billion annually in fundamental and applied research and technology development across a broad range of topics, including space and Earth sciences, life and physical sciences, human health, aeronautics, and technology (NASA 2014).

References

Gonzales, H. B. (2014). The National Science Foundation: Background and selected policy issues. *Congressional Research Service, 7–5700, Technical Report R43585.*

Mather, M., & Fanselow, M. S. (2018). Editorial overview: Interactions between emotion and cognition. *Current Opinion in Behavioral Sciences, 19,* iv–vi.

NASA. (2014). Plan for increasing access to the results of scientific research. Report to Office of Science and Technology Policy on November 21, 2014. Downloaded Nov, 8, 2016 from https://www.nasa.gov/sites/default/files/atoms/files/206985_2015_nasa_plan-for-web.pdf+&cd=2&hl=en&ct=clnk&gl=us

Okon-Singer, H. (2018). The role of attention bias to threat in anxiety: Mechanisms, modulators and open questions. *Current Opinion in Behavioral Sciences, 19,* 26–30.

von Hippel, T., & von Hippel, C. (2015). To apply or not to apply: A survey analysis of grant writing costs and benefits. *PLoS One, 10*(3), e0118494 Published online 2015 Mar. https://doi.org/10.1371/journal.pone.0118494.

Chapter 7
Funding Institution Vetting

We introduced the notion of vetting as a means of separating the impartial review of technical merit (peer review) from the process of evaluating the value of each favorably-scored project relative to the institution's mission, budget, and how the science complements its current grant or contract portfolio. Where vetting becomes an artform is when technical merit scores are in a fundable range, but the number of meritorious applications exceeds available funds. That is when shrewd applicants can game the system somewhat by reducing project costs or by obtaining outside funding from other ICs, agencies, foundations or even your own institution. Thus, understanding the vetting stage of grantsmanship can help you develop strategies for moving from the deferred category to the funded category.

7.1 Funding Plan

Funding Plan

- PO Recommendation
- Branch Nomination
- Division Short List
- Agency/Inst. Proposal
- Council Approval

As mentioned in the beginning of the chapter, NIH uses a two-level review system. Many funding institutions use only one. Once NIH peer review is completed, your application goes from "Initial Review" to "Secondary Review." That starts the

© The Author(s), under exclusive license to Springer Nature Switzerland AG 2019   91
T. F. Hilton, C. G. Leukefeld, *Grantsmanship for New Investigators*,
SpringerBriefs in Public Health, https://doi.org/10.1007/978-3-030-01301-1_7

vetting process. Basically, vetting is the process of assembling the IC's final Funding Plan to submit to its National Advisory Council for ratification.

7.1.1 PO Recommendations

The vetting process begins with POs determining which grants best complement their portfolios. They assemble a list of projects to consider for award and submit it to their Branch Chief. Each Branch whittles down their list before submitting their Funding Plan to their Division. Each Division Director, in turn, consolidates their plan in a meeting with the other Division Directors and the IC Director to consolidate the IC's formal Funding Plan for submission to their National Advisory Council for ratification. Throughout the process, POs might be requested to defend their recommendation for one or more grants – even before Council. While POs do not make the final award decision, they surely can have a lot of influence on the process.

The PO's recommendation decision is based on several factors:

1. Peer review score. If the score is quite low, and your relative percentile is low, then you are likely to get funded unless your project's costs are higher than normal for the funding mechanism (type of grant) applied for. That is why you are required to get permission to submit grants with budgets outside published guidelines.
2. Percentile. Percentiles are about competition. A score of 23 in one review session might be a 19 in another. Yet, that 23 might be in the 19th percentile, whereas the 19 might be in the 23rd percentile. Percentiles help when the list gets down to the proverbial wire when deciding which of the remaining meritorious grants will be recommended for award. In cases of low score but moderate percentile, your PO might encourage deferral because other projects assigned to the division will take precedence for the current cycle.
3. Budget. If your technical merit score is in a fundable range, but the project is quite costly, deferral might be considered. Deferral enables your PO to shop your project around to potential co-sponsors in order to lower the cost to the IC or decide to wait out another cycle to see if more funds will be available next quarter. How does deferral work? During every cycle, a variable number of old grants end, thereby freeing up additional funds for new projects. The next cycle's applications might not be as meritorious, or other institutions have decided to chip in as co-sponsors, and your deferred grant gets funding.
4. The summary statement. If, when identified weaknesses are examined, they are easily remedied prior to award, your grant might be a candidate for funding in the current or next funding cycle. If your project is a top mission priority, you might just get the benefit of the doubt as long as you are flexible and agree to minor changes.
5. The review meeting itself. If the PO attended, there might have been mitigating issues that in the PO's mind merited a better score. That might keep your application on the list if the PO can convince the Branch Chief and Division Director of

the value added by your project. This is usually the case when the project is cutting-edge or will help close an important knowledge gap in the branch portfolio.

6. Project importance. If your project addresses one or more designated high-priority topics, that too might keep it on the funding recommendation list as long as weaknesses can be easily remedied such as sample size, analyses, or missing information that can be amended during vetting.

7. Urgency. It sometimes makes little practical sense to wait the 6–9 months that it takes to revise-and-resubmit just to improve a fixable project with high mission urgency. If you as PI are willing to make some recommended changes on the spot, your PO might be able to keep your project on the list to get your award issued in the current cycle.

8. Portfolio alignment. If your project is not substantially different from projects already in the program portfolio for the queue awaiting award, even with a relatively low score, there is a chance that it will drop off the list. The best option for the PI is to rework the application and submit it elsewhere.

7.1.2   Branch Funding Plans

The Branch Chief normally meets with their POs to select the applications that appear to be most competitive within the branch and division. The division's draft funding plan is in a confidential online file for all staff to examine at any time, so Branch Chiefs and POs know what the competition in their branch, division, and IC looks like.

7.1.3   Division Funding Plans

Branch Chiefs meet with their Division Director to present their recommended projects for inclusion in the Division funding plan. A considerable amount of horse-trading is not uncommon at these meetings. Give and take ensures that most high-priority projects in each branch get on the Division plan, and it acquaints the Division Director with rationales to defend recommendations at the Funding Plan meeting with the IC Director. As can be expected, each branch sees some of its nominated projects fall off the Funding Plan into the deferral pool.

7.1.4   Agency/Institution Final Funding Plan

The final IC funding plan is assembled during a meeting between the Institute Director and Division Directors. Just like the division-level funding plan meetings, Division Directors usually engage in some horse-trading to allow high priority projects to remain on the funding plan list while others are deferred until the next application cycle. The Institute Director always makes the final decision on funding plans to be presented to the National Advisory Council. Again, more grants fall into the deferral pool.

7.1.5 Advisory Council Funding Plan Approval

Every federal and most private-sector funding institutions have advisory councils or boards comprised of leaders in the field, members of the public, and select stakeholders. At NIH, one should expect to see healthcare providers and leaders of various patient advocacy groups in addition to leading researchers. Each NIH IC has its own Council that meets at the end of each funding cycle (2–4 times a year). These councils serve several functions, not the least of which is to deflect political heat in event somebody in Congress takes issue with a funding decision. The primary role of Councils is to advise on policy matters and future directions. Included in the Council advisory role at NIH is ratification of funding plans.

NIH Councils hold two separate, back-to-back meetings. The first meeting is a session open to the press and public (space-permitting) during which council is briefed by IC leadership on progress with previously recommended initiatives, and council members (sometimes members of the public) suggest emergent needs for new studies and various initiatives aimed at enhancing mission accomplishment.

The second meeting is closed to the public. This is when the Funding Plan is presented and discussed Division by Division. At this meeting, the Division Director, Branch Chief, and possibly the PO might be engaged by the Council to defend recommendations. If the case is not made, the project is removed from the funding plan. Once each Division has presented its recommended portfolio, Council members may raise concerns or even encouragement regarding specific studies. Subsequently, a vote is cast for the entire proposed list on the Division funding plan (minus any projects Council rejects), and the award process begins.

7.2 The Award Process

Award Process

- Funding List
- Grants Management
- Pre-Award Negotiation
- Award Notice

- Renewal Application/ Progress Report

Because agencies want the best research for the taxpayers' money, they **strive to balance the amount of money spent against the number and diversity of projects supported**. For example, instead of funding one five-year $6 M grant – two dissertations, one two-year post-doc, and three smaller three-year research projects could be supported. Clearly, the apparent value of the big five-year project must justify its value added to the IC's portfolio if it is to be funded. The likelihood that all six smaller competing projects will fail is not only low, but unlikely to be noticed by the press. On the other hand, a failed $6 M project might generate a headline such as *"Six-Million-Dollar Project at State University Bombs While Tuition For 100 Students Goes Unfunded."* On the other hand, the greater the positive attention to everybody if project results justify the $6 M investment and the headline reads: *"Six-Million-Dollar Project at State University Discovers Promising Treatment for Cancer."*

Based upon what we have said, **the higher the cost of the proposed project**:

1. The more scrutiny it will get during peer review. Consequently:

   - The stronger the scientific case must be
   - The greater is the perceived benefit to the taxpayers
   - The more aims should be aligned with funding institution goals and priorities
   - The more experienced the proposed PI and research team should be
   - The more assets the proposed PI's institution should commit to
   - The more letters of cooperation from data and support sources should be included

2. The higher the risk of funding deferral (i.e., delay) because:

   - The longer it will take the Project Officer to make a case for funding
   - The higher the priority that project must have with the funding institution director
   - The more time it might take to get co-funding from other agencies and possibly foundations to lower the cost to the parent funding institution

3. The more likely that funding will be questioned by a federal agency's National Advisory Council.
4. If an award is made,

   - The more likely that multiple funding agencies and/or foundations will be involved.
   - The more carefully the Project Officer will monitor progress.

On the other hand, if an application is funded after passing through multiple layers of review, the odds are favorable that something very useful from the costly study will result from the project.

7.2.1   Funding List

The Funding List is just another term for the ratified Funding Plan. Once your application is on the Funding List, that *Train of Thought* you crafted has put your project
on track for a grant award. However, you are not quite yet at the desired destination.
As previously noted, the amount of your award may not be quite as generous as your
request, and some changes in your research plan may need to be made.

Much of the application's adjustment was likely completed before Council met
in order to maximize competitiveness. However, there are Federal rules and regulations that might require further adjustments, and your institution's grants office will
have to negotiate adjustments with the IC Grants Management Office to conform to
government rules and regulations.

7.2.2   Grants Management

Once Council has reviewed your application and it appears on the IC's final funding
plan, your application will be assigned a Grants Management Officer (GMO) –
another player with fate control. The IC's Grants Management Office is the central
clearing house for award negotiation, progress reports, and any fiscal problems that
might arise for which your grant requires IC approval (normally via your PO). You
might think of your GMO as the funding institution's CPA.

Your GMO is responsible for pre-award negotiation with your institutions (See
the next Section), and ensures compliance with all laws, rules, and regulations for
the life of your grant. In addition, suppose you discover that one arm of your study
appears to be harmful to subjects, or you get access to new technology and want to
change a service contract. Your PO and GMO are the people with whom to work in
order to coordinate these kinds of changes. Your GMO is not always the approval
authority. Anything related to your research plan or progress will require prior PO
approval to insure research integrity. For now, at this stage of funding, the GMO is
the person who will finalize the terms of grant award or contract amount for your
approved application.

7.2.3   Pre-award Negotiation

Nearly all applications involve some negotiation with the applicant institution. In
some cases, your institution may be requesting direct costs which are already
included in the established indirect cost rate and are not allowed by law; or they may
be including salaries over the NIH salary cap. There also might be research plan
changes that will affect costs, and that will have to be amended to reflect new costs.
Usually, this is a painless process, and you as PI or fellowship awardee might not
even be involved. That is because your institution is technically the awardee, and as
such, is legally on the hook for compliance with the terms of award.

7.2.4   Award Notice

Once your GMO and, you, and your AOR have an agreed upon the budget, and all required training, certifications, and other requirements have been submitted and accepted; you will get a preliminary **Notice of Grant Award (NGA).** The NIH Grants Policy Statement stipulates the conditions of all NIH grants except as amended by your specific NGA. Once the preliminary NGA is accepted by your AOR, you will receive an email from NIH that constitutes the official Notice of Grant (or Contract) Award. You may now, start spending federal money on your project.

But wait a minute! **Who pays for pre-award costs?** Perhaps your institution spent almost $9,000 before the award in order to reserve access to equipment, a laboratory, or office space, for example. Who pays for that? The applying institution absorbs all costs associated with its grant applications. You may not charge those costs to your first-year budget. Of course, most grants include an institutional and indirect costs rate (overhead), so your institution is only technically out-of-pocket. **Who pays for pre-award costs if you do not get a grant or contract?** Maybe you did not score competitively, or somewhere along the line, your application got bumped off the pay list. In any case, the answer is the same. Your institutional overhead absorbs the cost – your time and pay are not compensated directly. However, most faculty are salaried; not paid by the hours worked.

7.3   Progress Reports

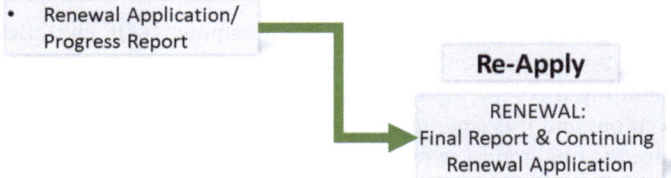

Virtually all funding institutions require progress reports and final reports. NIH Progress reports (PHS 2590) are normally submitted annually 6–8 weeks before the end of each award year unless more frequent reports are stipulated in your NGA. Complex projects may require more frequent updates, either formally or over the phone. Progress reports basically summarize who did what, for how much, and to whom. Most federal agency progress reports are submitted on line by your institution's AOR unless delegated to you.

When your progress report arrives at the funding institution, the GMO will focus in on your budget summary, whereas your PO, for example, is likely to focus on the diversity of your recruiting and the number of subjects enrolled and under study. The reason POs focus on recruiting progress is simple. This phase is where many projects involving human subjects lose ground and milestones start to slip. When that happens your funding institution risks having to supplement your award with additional funds to ensure project completion. That is not desirable. Alternatively, you normally apply for a "no-cost" extension as long as there are un-committed funds remaining in your award account.

Your professional life will be less stressful if you focus on getting your sample recruited and enrolled as stipulated in your application schedule. In the middle phase of your project, once subjects are being exposed to the experimental condition(s), PO attention shifts to human subject retention, animal survival, and adverse events. After all, a large drop in follow-up data affects power and the validity of outcomes.

There are ways to engage study participants at the recruitment phase that will improve retention at follow-up(s). It requires a bit more planning up-front and identifying clever incentives for staying engaged with subjects. Again, we recommend reading Scott (2004) before you draft your research plan. Scott's research team consistently achieves high levels of retention (>90%) over several years' duration among drug addicts, a population that is about as difficult to track as the Abominable Snowman.

7.4   Final Reports and Competing Renewal Applications

Final Reports By law, all federally-funded research requires at least one tangible deliverable. A final report is always due within 90 days of project termination. The final report summarizes what went on in the project, discusses findings, and clarifies what was learned or discovered.

Competing Renewals Eventually, your grant support will end. Before you reach that milestone, you should decide whether or not you can make a strong case for submitting a competing continuation application; or whether your data mine is played out and it is time to summarize achievements and move on. Most NIH ICs waive the final report requirement if you are competing for grant renewal because the application includes accomplishments from the previous project grant. Until recently, NIH made it essential that any continuing application include a radical departure – innovation – from the hypotheses previously under study, even though the project may have at best harvested half a loaf during its lifespan. In recent years that requirement has been relaxed. You will probably be competitive if you make a solid case that continued research will add or extend knowledge, and that your team's experience and expertise is well-suited to continue harvesting that useful knowledge. If your original application suggested that possibility – all the better.

Competing Renewal Timing If it looks like there remains a significant amount of scientific gold *in them thar hills*, you should start talking with your PO about 18 months before your RPG's funding is due to end. You want to start considering ways to make your competing continuation application "competitive," and to establish optimal timing for your new submission. There are two possible scenarios for timing the submission of a **Competing Continuation (Renewal) Application**. Some investigators prefer to have the application reviewed and approved by Council just before the current grant award ends, so there is no lapse in funding. However, many projects encounter delays, and will be completing data analyses and writing reports for several months after the end of the award period. As mentioned earlier, in those cases, PIs request a **no-cost extension** from their PO and schedule submission of their competing renewal application accordingly. Extension approval is normally perfunctory which allows you to continue to spend residual funds remaining in the grant for up to 12 months.

<u>Final Report Content</u> At NIH, and many other federal funding institutions, sophisticated data systems have been developed to monitor progress in order to maintain accountability to Congress and the American public. Thus, for these agencies, final reports have become perfunctory, and may seldom be read by anybody unless part of a competing renewal application. However, **many foundations still place considerable value in them** as justification for their investments. Thus, those reports are often presented to foundation board members. Likewise, contracts might stipulate a final report as a required deliverable.

Unless yours is a short project, your application aims section, prior progress reports, and any draft publications should enable you to cut and paste a reasonably hefty report in short order that meets guidelines. Make sure all accomplishments are listed because **you never know who might dredge up this very public document** in the future as part of an investigation by the press, Congress, or a state official.

That brings us to the end of the application and award cycle. It will be up to you when that cycle will end. If your research career is successful, it will likely end when some life event, or maybe even a plan, triggers your retirement. Good luck!

Reference

Scott, C. K. (2004). A replicable model for achieving over 90% follow-up rates in longitudinal studies of substance abusers. *Drug and Alcohol Dependence, 74*(2004), 21–36.

Closing Remarks

Throughout this book, our focus has been on providing sufficient information for you to decide if grants or contracts are appropriate ways for you to build your academic research career. We introduced you to the basic elements of a successful application or contract proposal and described in general terms how grants and contracts are reviewed and vetted. Our goal has been to enable you to apply tactics and strategies (*grantsmanship*) that will enhance the likelihood of receiving an award to support your research throughout your career.

The very word *grantsmanship* is open to diverse interpretations. Wikipedia defines *grantsmanship* as "the art of acquiring peer-reviewed research funding." Of course, defining grantsmanship as an art suggests that success hinges mainly on innate talent like a Da Vinci painting, a Michelangelo sculpture or I. M. Pei architecture. The term also includes the term "man," which might suggest that there is a "good-ole-boy" network involved. As a researcher, you are part of that network. Art also connotes an evolving skill, which grantsmanship certainly is. A good-ole-boy network also suggests that personal relationships trump merit. However, attributing competitive failure to an unfair system (of which you are a part) merely saves face and relegates *grantsmanship* to gambling, which it is not.

As we mentioned, a record of accomplishment does give seasoned grantees a competitive edge, but not because of who they know; but what they have learned. From what we have observed over a combined period spanning more than 80 years is that strategic thinking and hard work are far more essential to successful *grantsmanship* than any of the negative connotations mentioned.

We hope that we have made it clear that *grantsmanship* is not just about submitting a competitive application. It is a collaborative effort between you and your mentors, colleagues and your project team; your institution; and not infrequently, your target funding institution and other interested funders. Even after your project is reviewed and scored, there are things that you can do to make your project more competitive – including revising and resubmitting your application.

101
T. F. Hilton, C. G. Leukefeld, *Grantsmanship for New Investigators*,
SpringerBriefs in Public Health, https://doi.org/10.1007/978-3-030-01301-1

In closing, we want to remind you that grantsmanship is a developmental process. Both you and the grant environment are always evolving. Thus, continue reading about changes in the priorities and procedures of your target funding institutions, like keeping up with the changing literature in your scientific field. It will help to ensure continued support for your research projects during your entire career. We talk a bit more at length about this topic in Appendix C and offer some helpful hyperlinks. We wish you the best success in your research career and hope that in some way our book will help you stay on that path to success.

Reference

Wikipedia (2017). Grantsmanship. Downloaded on June 06, 2017 from: https://en.wikipedia.org/wiki/Grantsmanship

Appendix A: NIH Research Project Grant Initial Review Criteria

A.1 Significance

Does the project address an important problem or a critical barrier to progress in the field? Is there a strong scientific premise for the project? If the aims of the project are achieved, how will scientific knowledge, technical capability, and/or clinical practice be improved? How will successful completion of the aims change the concepts, methods, technologies, treatments, services, or preventative interventions that drive this field?

A.2 Investigator(s)

Are the PIs, Co-I's, collaborators, and other researchers well suited to the project? If Early Stage Investigators or New Investigators, or in the early stages of independent careers, do they have appropriate experience and training? If established, have they demonstrated an ongoing record of accomplishments that have advanced their field(s)? If the project is collaborative or multi-PI, do the investigators have complementary and integrated expertise; are their leadership approach, governance and organizational structure appropriate for the project?

A.3 Innovation

Does the application challenge and seek to shift current research or clinical practice paradigms by utilizing novel theoretical concepts, approaches or methodologies, instrumentation, or interventions? Are the concepts, approaches or methodologies,

© The Author(s), under exclusive license to Springer Nature Switzerland AG 2019
T. F. Hilton, C. G. Leukefeld, *Grantsmanship for New Investigators*,
SpringerBriefs in Public Health, https://doi.org/10.1007/978-3-030-01301-1

instrumentation, or interventions novel to one field of research or novel in a broad sense? Is a refinement, improvement, or new application of theoretical concepts, approaches or methodologies, instrumentation, or interventions proposed?

A.4 Approach

Are the overall strategy, methodology, and analyses well-reasoned and appropriate to accomplish the specific aims of the project? Have the investigators presented strategies to ensure a robust and unbiased approach, as appropriate for the work proposed? Are potential problems, alternative strategies, and benchmarks for success presented? If the project is in the early stages of development, will the strategy establish feasibility and will particularly risky aspects be managed? Have the investigators presented adequate plans to address relevant biological variables, such as sex, for studies in vertebrate animals or human subjects?

If the project involves human subjects and/or NIH-defined clinical research, are the plans to address 1) the protection of human subjects from research risks, and 2) the inclusion (or exclusion) of individuals on the basis of sex/gender, race, and ethnicity, as well as the inclusion (exclusion) of children, justified in terms of the scientific goals and research strategy proposed?

A.5 Environment

Will the scientific environment in which the work will be done contribute to the probability of success? Are the institutional support, equipment and other physical resources available to the investigators adequate for the project proposed? Will the project benefit from unique features of the scientific environment, subject populations, or collaborative arrangements?

Appendix B: Review Criteria for Regulatory Compliance

Protections for Human Subjects, Vertebrate Animals, and Biohazards
These all represent potential showstoppers in review because in the majority of cases your application will require revision before it can receive a score.

- If proposing a clinical trial, a data and safety monitoring plan (DSMP) must be included. Guidelines are available for DSMPs on NIH websites.
- If using animals, explain why you are using animals vs human subjects and defend your selection of species to study. For example, if most studies have been using Norwegian rats, explain why your study is using stray cats.

Inclusion of Women, Minorities and Children
This topic must be addressed in all applications involving Human Subjects. Skipping this topic in an application because the disease under study normally afflicts one group (e.g., breast cancer) is a mistake. Explain why your sample does not include other groups or expect a higher score.

B.1 Additional Review Considerations

B.1.1 Applications from Foreign Organizations

Applications from foreign organizations must present special opportunities for furthering research programs through the use of unusual talent, resources, populations, or environmental conditions unique to the applicant's country. That is, they either are not readily available in the United States or augment existing U.S. resources.

© The Author(s), under exclusive license to Springer Nature Switzerland AG 2019
T. F. Hilton, C. G. Leukefeld, *Grantsmanship for New Investigators*,
SpringerBriefs in Public Health, https://doi.org/10.1007/978-3-030-01301-1

B.1.2 Biological Select Agents or Toxins

Reviewers will assess the information provided in this section of the application, including (1) the Select Agent(s) or toxins to be used in the proposed research, (2) the registration status of all entities where Select Agent(s) will be used, (3) the procedures that will be used to monitor possession use and transfer of Select Agent(s), and (4) plans for appropriate biosafety, biocontainment, and security of the Select Agent(s). Any omissions or vague descriptions will result in an unfundable score.

B.1.3 Resource Sharing Plans

You must include a Resource Sharing Plan or provide a rationale for not sharing your data. Keep in mind that your plan does not undermine patient privacy or other human subject vulnerabilities.

B.1.4 Authentication of Key Biological and/or Chemical Resources

For projects involving key biological and/or chemical resources, comment on the brief plans proposed for identifying and ensuring the validity of those resources.

Appendix C: Funding Institution Interests

Applicants take a big risk when trying to pursue projects that seem to be "hot" at the moment. Nevertheless, all agencies have **emergent** AND **standing** priorities. If your lab is already tooled up to jump on an emergent crisis – then by all means go for it. In most cases, the standing priorities are still your best bet.

Nearly all federal agencies publish their priorities. Alas, they are often broadly written and offer little insight about what the agency really wants. For example, most NIH Program Announcements almost read like "Guess what we want to fund." That is where agency program staff can be helpful. Every PO has a matrix of possibilities they would like to see in the portfolios they administer. You are likely to be more successful if a program or project staff member is eager to see your project in their portfolio. Keep in mind that it is the PO who is responsible for getting research completed for public health, national defense, public safety needs, etc.

POs have an understanding of the big picture as it applies to research. Not only do they sit on National Advisory Council meetings, they sit in on most peer review meetings, and listen to the give and take between leaders in their field as they discuss applications, and regularly attend NIH symposia presented by world leaders in their field.

Another helpful source of information about grant priorities comes from program announcements, requests for proposals, agency plans, email and word of mouth.

Identifying Areas of Interest

http://grants.nih.gov/grants/guide/pa-files/index.html
http://nsf.gov/funding/
https://www.onr.navy.mil/Contracts-Grants/Funding-Opportunities

- Primary portal for all **grant** applications: https://www.grants.gov/ OR
- Primary portal for all federal **contracts** is FedBizOps: https://www.fbo.gov/ index?s=main&mode=list&tab=list

© The Author(s), under exclusive license to Springer Nature Switzerland AG 2019   107
T. F. Hilton, C. G. Leukefeld, *Grantsmanship for New Investigators*,
SpringerBriefs in Public Health, https://doi.org/10.1007/978-3-030-01301-1

Looking for COLLABORATORS? Want to know who in your university, city, or state is doing work in your area? Want to find colleagues working in the same area of interest? Search https://projectreporter.nih.gov/reporter.cfm

Overviews most NSF Grant processes: https://www.nsf.gov/funding/preparing/

Appendix D: Outline for a Grant or Contract Letter of Support

Opening Paragraph

- LOS Writer's role/title; institution/organization (Chair, Department of Engineering, University X; Senior Key personnel on the project)
- Why they are writing?

  – To support the proposal or agree to participate (advisory board, preceptor, etc.)
  – To commit resources
  – To provide cost share/matching funds

- Proposal identifier

  – Project Title
  – Grant number (only if a revision)
  – Type of grant (e.g., R01, K23, P01)

Body Paragraph(s)

- Overview perceived project strengths

  – Scientific plan/your own fit in the project, if participating/advisory board
  – Proposal leadership
  – Team of scientists/staff
  – Mentorship (if applicable)
  – Track record of publications or training of proposal PI

- Briefly describe institutional strengths relevant to proposal

  – Proposal aligns with organization strategic plan
  – Leadership/faculty expertise
  – Resources/facilities for the project
  – Achievements that demonstrate high caliber

© The Author(s), under exclusive license to Springer Nature Switzerland AG 2019
T. F. Hilton, C. G. Leukefeld, *Grantsmanship for New Investigators*,
SpringerBriefs in Public Health, https://doi.org/10.1007/978-3-030-01301-1

- If relevant, specifically outline commitment – what their organization is contributing (Include rate/charge for any services)

- What are they contributing to the project (e.g., time, resources, analyses, assays, fabrication, code writing – the more specific; the better)?
- Experience & expertise

Concluding Paragraph/Close

Appendix E: Acronyms Used in Grants/Contracts Administration

AE	Adverse Event
AOR	AOR (Authorized Organization Representative) – aka Signing Official
AREA	Academic Research Enhancement Award
ARF/ PHS-ARF	Assignment Request Form used to indicate a peer review panel preference
BAA	Broad Area Announcement (contract or grant opportunity; also RFP, RFA, FOA, PA)
CO	Contracting Officer
CO-I	Co-Investigator, a collaborating colleague of any academic rank. Co-Is are not PIs
CO-PI	Co-principal Investigator (NIH only recognizes one PI/grant. Co-PI is thus a Co-I)
COTR	Contracting Officer's Technical Representative (Usually a scientist)
CSR	Center for Scientific Review
DSMB	Data & Safety Monitoring Board
DSMP	Data & Safety Monitoring Plan
DSP/DSRP	Data Sharing Plan / Data & Resource Sharing Plan (For GWAS projects)
ERC	European Research Council
ESI	Early Stage Investigator
FOA	Funding Opportunity Announcement
FWA	Federalwide Assurance
GAO	Government Accountability Office
GMO	Grants Management Officer (oversees compliance with regulations)
GWAS	Genome-wide Association Study (study involving the human genome)
HS	Human Subjects
IC	Institute/Center (refers to NIH institutes)
IRB	Institutional Review Board
IRG	Initial Review Group, also Study Section, also peer review panel

(continued)

(continued)

LOE	Level Of Effort
LOS	Letter of Support
ND or NS	Not Discussed also NS (not scored)
NDA	Nondisclosure Agreement
NGA	Notice of Grant Award (formal grant award)
NI	New Investigator
NRFC	Not Recommended For Further Consideration (banned from re-application)
OBE	Overcome By Events
PA	Program Announcement (NIH or NSF standing FOA)
PD	Program Director (Develops and administers portfolio of grants in specified areas)
PDW	Professional Development Workshop
PHS	Public Health Service
PI	Principal Investigator
PO	Project Officer
PO	Program Official (Develops and administers portfolio of grants in specified areas)
R&D	Research and Development
RFA	Request for Applications (special grant announcement)
RFP	Request for Proposals (type of contract announcement)
RPG	Research Project Grant
SAE	Serious Adverse Event
SBIR	Small Business Innovation Research grant
SO	Science Officer (government-assigned co-investigator/Co-I)
SRO	Scientific Review Officer (coordinates peer reviews)
STTR	Small Business Technology Transfer Research grant
TBA	To Be Assigned/Arranged (some post-award activity)

Note: List does not include federal departments and agency abbreviations

Index

© The Author(s), under exclusive license to Springer Nature Switzerland AG 2019   113
T. F. Hilton, C. G. Leukefeld, *Grantsmanship for New Investigators*,
SpringerBriefs in Public Health, https://doi.org/10.1007/978-3-030-01301-1